SpringerBriefs in Well-Being and Quality of Life Research

More information about this series at http://www.springer.com/series/10150

Liora Findler · Orit Taubman – Ben-Ari

Grandparents of Children with Disabilities

Theoretical Perspectives of Intergenerational Relationships

with Shirley Ben Shlomo and Adi Noy

Springer

Liora Findler
The Louis and Gabi Weisfeld School of Social Work
Bar-Ilan University
Ramat-Gan
Israel

Orit Taubman – Ben-Ari
The Louis and Gabi Weisfeld School of Social Work
Bar-Ilan University
Ramat-Gan
Israel

ISSN 2211-7644 ISSN 2211-7652 (electronic)
SpringerBriefs in Well-Being and Quality of Life Research
ISBN 978-3-319-45515-0 ISBN 978-3-319-45517-4 (eBook)
DOI 10.1007/978-3-319-45517-4

Library of Congress Control Number: 2016949565

Printed on acid-free paper

This Springer imprint is published by Springer Nature
The registered company is Springer International Publishing AG
The registered company address is: Gewerbestrasse 11, 6330 Cham, Switzerland

Foreword

This is an important book. It is about grandparenting, a topic which has only recently gotten the attention it deserves from social scientists. Moreover, it is about grandparents of children with disabilities, a situation which has received almost no attention by scholars to date. And finally it is about theory, about how and why grandparents do what they do with grandchildren who are significantly challenged.

Grandparenthood is one of the most significant social roles of later life. It is also one of the least charted. What should we do as a grandparent, or what should we not do? It is a role that is thrust upon us; we have no way to become grandparents except through the actions of our children when they become parents. Grandparenthood is a complex enterprise that provides both opportunities and challenges and joys and concerns, and we have few cultural guidelines in our society that help us negotiate these issues.

The situation of grandparents involved in the lives of grandchildren with disabilities poses additional complexities. Very little research until now has addressed this issue, and the chapters in this volume make an important advancement in knowledge. Here, we learn about the instrumental and emotional support that can be provided by grandparents and the factors contributing to, or inhibiting, their role in the lives of grandchildren with disabilities. The authors report results from an innovative study that examines, for the first time, the possibilities for positive outcomes and personal growth among grandparents of children with disabilities. This documents the unique contributions of grandparents to the parents' own adjustment to this new reality—that their child has a disability—and how they might negotiate the delicate balance between helping and intruding.

Grandparents of Children with Disabilities is a milestone in the literature on families and is unique by tapping an issue that is a part of our lives, yet is almost overlooked in the professional literature. It is also unique because it combines theory and research with the voices of grandmothers and grandfathers.

This book advances theory, about how and why grandparents do what they do with grandchildren who are significantly challenged. Almost all of the research literature to date has been descriptive, reporting on numbers of grandparents, what they do, describing the characteristics of relationships with grandchildren. The authors have gone beyond description to address the how and why of these relationships. The opening chapter is rich with theoretical insights such as these, and the subsequent chapters build upon theory to provide understanding.

Grandparents of Children with Disabilities will be a valuable source for professionals in various disciplines such as psychology, education, social work, and medicine, all working with families. It is written in a friendly way and can be an enriching source for family members in general and parents and grandparents in particular.

I hope that this book will raise the awareness of professionals to the unique and complex role of grandparents and will lead to changes in family-therapy perceptions, to more interventions with grandparents and to the inclusion of all generations in their professional activities.

Vern L. Bengtson
University of Southern California

Contents

About the Authors

Prof. Liora Findler is the head of the Rehabilitation and Health Track at the Louis and Gabi Weisfeld School of Social Work at Bar-Ilan University in Israel, and formerly headed Social Work services at the Child Development Center in Northern Israel. She specializes in families of children with disabilities and their intergenerational relations in particular, with an emphasis on positive outcomes and personal growth alongside the challenges and difficulties. Much of her research focuses on the unique experience of grandparents in these families, an area in which she is an internationally recognized expert.

Prof. Orit Taubman – Ben-Ari is a psychologist and professor at the Louis and Gabi Weisfeld School of Social Work at Bar-Ilan University in Israel. For the past fifteen years, she has studied intergenerational relationships and personal growth following life transitions, such as the transitions to parenthood and grandparenthood. In the wake of her ground-breaking research, her scholarly publications were among the first to introduce the construct of personal growth into the discourse of life transitions. Her studies examine both deleterious and positive or constructive predispositions and outcomes within families coping with various stress-related events, and she has published extensively on these issues in international journals.

Dr. Shirley Ben Shlomo is a clinical social worker and psychotherapist specializing in parents, children, and youth. She is a lecturer and the head of the Bachelor's degree program at the Louis and Gabi Weisfeld School of Social Work at Bar-Ilan University in Israel. Her research focuses on positive outcomes following life transitions, the representation of social work in the media, and developmental implications of intergenerational transmission of abuse and neglect. Her papers have been published in scientific journals and presented at international conferences.

Dr. Adi Noy is a clinical social worker and lecturer at the Louis and Gabi Weisfeld School of Social Work at Bar-Ilan University in Israel. She specializes in children and adolescents with psychological and behavioral difficulties and is currently working at the child and youth clinic in Shalvata Psychiatric Hospital. Her Ph.D. focused on the transition to motherhood, taking into account intergenerational relationships with grandparents. Her research has been published in scientific journals and presented at international conferences.

Introduction: On Adding "Grand" to Parenthood

Liora Findler and Orit Taubman - Ben-Ari

Grandparents are often surprised when they are approached by researchers or clinicians. Indeed, in response to our request to interview them for a study on intergenerational relations in families of children with disabilities, many grandparents wondered: "Why are you interested in us?"; "What do we matter?"; or "Why are you asking us and not our children?" But their surprise quickly gave way to an eagerness to open up and share their experience, and the dialogue that ensued revealed an intricate web of joy, pain, strain, satisfaction, and disappointment. An urge to discuss the grandparents was also evidenced by their children, the parents of a child with a disability. Time and time again, interviews with this middle generation provoked reference to the function of the grandparents in the family, the sensitivity and emotionality of their relationship with them, their expectations from each other, and the avenues of communication between them.

Grandparenthood is one of the most significant family roles in later life. Yet it is a status that is "born," without any choice on the part of the grandparent or any ability to control its timing, and the individual playing this role is not the featured actor on the stage. Moreover, the frequency of meetings with the grandchild, the degree of involvement in their life, and the nature of the relationship with them is determined largely by their children, that is, the grandchild's parents, and not by the grandparents alone. But alongside the lack of control and the possibility of unmet expectations, playing a secondary role, has certain advantages, such as freedom from direct responsibility for raising the child, the chance to experience a more mature model of parenthood, and the luxury of simply enjoying and pampering the child without always having to exert authority and set boundaries.

Grandparenthood is thus a complex experience that poses considerable challenges which raise questions about the role and status of the grandparents from numerous angles. The parents' discourse on grandparents runs the gamut from gratitude for their help and contribution to the family to a view of them as a burden, from the expectation of receiving emotional, instrumental, and financial support to a fear of their interference, from the desire for their advice to a dread of criticism.

The increase in longevity in recent decades has created a new reality in which three, or even four, generations may live together for many years. At the same time, social change has generated new family models, including single-parent and single-sex families, which also impact the nature of intergenerational relationships and the role of the grandparents. Moreover, this role is affected by the personalities of the family members, the structure and character of the family, and the social and cultural context. In addition, over the course of time, family relations are influenced by crises or changes both in society and in the family itself, painting intergenerational relationships in new and different colors.

If this compound reality constitutes a challenge in "typical" families, it goes without saying that coping with it is even more challenging for families in special circumstances, such as those experiencing divorce, death, disability, or illness. While this book is dedicated primarily to grandparents in families of a child with a disability, it also relates to the role and meaning of grandparenthood in any family. In fact, a special chapter is devoted to becoming a grandparent, a normative life transition that has received little attention in the clinical and empirical literature.

Despite the growing presence of grandparents in the therapeutic discourse with parents of children with disabilities, reference to the place and function of the grandparents in such families is conspicuous by its absence from clinical, research, and theoretical literature. This book is aimed at filling that gap by turning the spotlight on grandparents and intergenerational relationships in families of children with disabilities, offering the perspectives of grandparents, parents, and professionals.

Chapter 1, written by Dr. Shirley Ben Shlomo and Prof. Orit Taubman – Ben-Ari, charts the historical development of research and theory on grandparenthood and presents the contemporary theoretical approaches to the concept and role of grandparents. The chapter stresses the need to understand the complexity of grandparenthood in light of the increase in longevity and decrease in fertility and birth rate in modern society, which have made it one of the central and longest-held roles in an individual's life. Historical attitudes are examined in terms of social expectations and the relationship between grandparents and grandchildren, which may persist in the latter's adult life. The role is also discussed in relation to the emergence of specific sociodemographic and familial characteristics, such as the rise in the number of single-parent and single-sex families, which have created new patterns of intergenerational relationships. The chapter concludes with a discussion of the challenges facing future research.

Chapter 2, by Dr. Adi Noy and Prof. Orit Taubman – Ben-Ari, relates to the transition to grandparenthood. Although perceived as one of the most significant and emotional life events, it has only recently become the subject of comprehensive research. The chapter offers a wide view of this experience from the perspective of the life cycle and other transitions, surveying the various factors that shape the experience of grandparenthood, the psychological well-being of grandparents, and the process of personal growth (i.e., positive psychological change) that may be triggered by the new role.

Chapter 3, by Prof. Liora Findler, relates specifically to grandparents in families of children with disabilities, discussing adaptation to the role of grandparent in light of the grandchild's disability. The survey of the empirical and theoretical literature, along with the voices of grandparents themselves culled from interviews conducted with them, reveals their feelings, insights, and experiences in respect to their children and grandchildren. The chapter describes the instrumental and emotional support provided by the grandparents and the factors contributing to or inhibiting their involvement and/or interference in the life of the family. This is followed by an innovative study that examined, for the first time, the possibility of positive outcomes and personal growth among grandparents of children with disabilities.

Chapter 4, also by Prof. Liora Findler, examines the role of the grandparents of children with disabilities from the point of view of the parents, the middle generation. It describes the unique contribution of the grandparents to the parents' adjustment to their new reality, considering how each of the parents perceives the place of the grandfathers versus the grandmothers and the maternal grandparents versus the paternal grandparents. The chapter relates at length to the costs and benefits of the relationship with the grandparents, examining differences between the two generations in respect to expectations, channels of communication, and the provision or non-provision of support, as well as the parents' assessment of the quality of the grandparents' involvement.

Chapter 5, by Dr. Adi Noy and Prof. Liora Findler, deals with a phenomenon that has been growing in recent decades: grandparents raising a grandchild with a disability. These custodial grandparents take over the parental function, whether temporarily or permanently. Fulfilling the role of parent entails considerable burdens and has far-reaching implications on both the personal and interpersonal levels. The chapter describes the characteristics of custodial grandparents, as well as the particular needs arising from the task of raising a grandchild and the costs and benefits of the role. In addition, it discusses the ways in which these grandparents make use of community services and other formal sources of support.

Chapter 6, written by Prof. Liora Findler, relates to professionals' perspective on the role of the grandparents in families of children with disabilities, presenting an integrative survey of three studies that investigated the attitudes of different categories of professionals: social workers; educators (school and kindergarten teachers); and healthcare workers (pediatricians and nurses). Each of the studies examined perception of the importance of the support provided to the family by the grandparents, the type of support required by the parents, and the type of support provided in practice, along with assessment of the contribution of the grandparents' support to the parents' adjustment and the costs and benefits of the support received. In addition, the professionals were asked to describe how their perception of the grandparental role is expressed in their work with these families.

In these six chapters, we have sought to paint a broad and insightful picture of the experience of grandparents in general and grandparents of children with disabilities in particular. It is our aim here to enable a voice that is often silent to be heard, to give expression to grandparents' pain, disappointment, and frustration, as well as to their readiness to pitch in, their devotion to the family, and the deep satisfaction they derive from fulfilling their role in the course of life. We hope the book is merely the first step toward recognizing this unique voice, and that it will pave the way for greater attention to be paid to grandparents on the theoretical, empirical, and clinical levels.

We would like to express our gratitude to Esther Otten from Springer publication who recognized both the need and importance of publishing this book. We thank Esther and Hendrike Tuerlings for their professional and generous assistance throughout the writing process.

On a personal note, we would like to thank our own grandparents for the part they have played in our lives and those of our children. They have helped us understand our place in the world and served as role models, as well as being the source of an infinite experience of unconditional love. There is no doubt in our minds that without them we would not be who we are today and we would not have the same passionate desire to delve deeply into the subject of grandparenthood.

Liora Findler
Orit Taubman – Ben-Ari

Chapter 1
Grandparenthood—Grand Generativity

Shirley Ben Shlomo and Orit Taubman – Ben-Ari

Abstract Grandparenthood has gained enhanced importance in recent decades as a result of the increase in longevity and decrease in fertility and birth rate which have made it not only one of the most significant roles in an individual's life, but also one of the longest-held. This chapter presents a historical "road map" of the theoretical and empirical study of grandparenthood, beginning with a review of the various theoretical approaches. This is followed by a discussion of the definition of the grandparent role and a description of the relationship between grandparents and their grandchildren, with a focus on current trends in research. The role is also discussed in relation to the emergence of specific sociodemographic and familial characteristics, such as the rise in the number of single-parent and single-sex families, which have created new patterns of intergenerational relationships. The chapter concludes with a discussion of the challenges facing future research and clinical practice.

Keywords Grandparenthood · Grandparents · Grandchildren · Family · Role definition · Intergenerational relationship

Grandparenthood, one of the most significant roles in life (Smith 2002), has gained enhanced importance in recent decades as a result of two demographic trends in modern society. The first is increased longevity. Individuals who become grandparents in middle age now continue to fulfill the role through the young-old and even old-old years (Szinovacz 1998). In fact, in today's world, people are grandparents for an average of 25 years. Many live long enough to see their grandchildren become young adults, which means that grandchildren have grandparents in their lives throughout their childhood, adolescence, and young adulthood (Rossi and Rossi 1990; Silverstein and Long 1998). The second trend is the decline in fertility and birth rates due to personal choice (Johnson and Troll 1996). According to Bengston and Mangen (1988), increased longevity and decreased fertility have led to the "verticalization" of the family structure, that is, to an increase in the number of living generations and a decrease in the number of people within each generation.

L. Findler and O. Taubman – Ben-Ari, *Grandparents of Children with Disabilities*,
SpringerBriefs in Well-Being and Quality of Life Research,
DOI 10.1007/978-3-319-45517-4_1

The implications of these trends go beyond mere demographics. Family life itself has become multigenerational. The emphasis on education and career development has increased expectations from grandparents to help with childcare (e.g., Ben Shlomo and Taubman – Ben-Ari 2012), and longer life expectancy has obliged the middle and younger generations to take an active part in the care of their aging parents or grandparents. The change in family models, such as the rise in single parent and same-sex households, has also heightened expectations from grandparents to help with childcare (Mansson 2015; Szinovacz 1998), especially in the event of challenging circumstances such as teenage pregnancy. This situation may lead to the blurring of boundaries between generations (Lowenstein 2010), as well as greater stress in the multigenerational family resulting in a decrease in the well-being of the different family members. At the same time, however, it may offer opportunities for their growth and development.

The current chapter presents a historical "road map" of the theoretical and empirical study of grandparenthood, beginning with the various theoretical approaches. This is followed by a discussion of the definition of the grandparent role and a description of the relationship between grandparents and their grandchildren, with a focus on current research trends.

1.1 Development of the Concept of Grandparenthood

Until the 1980s, grandparenthood as a social and familial role was largely ignored, both in the theoretical and empirical literature and in clinical practice. Tinsley and Parke (1984) suggest possible explanations for this neglect, such as the limited role grandparents played in the lives of their grandchildren in previous centuries when life expectancy was lower, and the prevailing attitude that the family is a unit consisting only of parents and children. The same attitude was commonly adopted in regard to child development, which was perceived to be dependent solely on the parent-child dyad, without reference to others in the extended family. Methodological problems also impeded research. Many grandparents were old and/or sick, making them less suitable subjects for standard interviewing techniques. In addition, almost no statistical or theoretical models for the examination of complex intergenerational relationships were available.

The change in the scientific literature on grandparenthood that began in the 1980s was not only quantitative, but also qualitative. The first publications on the subject, which appeared in the 1930s and 1940s, had taken a negative view of grandparents. Vollmer (1937), cited in Smith (2002) for example, published a paper entitled "Grandmother: A problem in child rearing," and Rappaport (1958, in Miller and Sandberg 1998) characterized grandparents as being over-involved in the lives of their grandchildren, coining the expression "the grandparent syndrome". The 1960s to the 1980s saw a gradual shift toward a more positive perception of the grandparent role (Borenstein 2002), ultimately leading Barranti (1985) to use the phrase "family resource" in relation to grandparents, while Troll (1985) referred to them as the "family watchdog". Grandparents now came to be perceived as a central source of support for families in general, and grandchildren in particular, especially in times of crisis, such as divorce or parental dysfunction. This positive trend was enhanced by the development of family theories, which focused on the extended family rather than the nuclear family alone (Miller and Sandberg 1998). As we shall see below, each of the central theories in the social sciences that were developed around this time related to the issue of grandparenthood from its own distinct perspective.

1.2 Theoretical Approaches to Grandparenthood

Theories regarding grandparenthood and the relationship between grandparents and grandchildren can be divided into a number of different categories, including evolutionary and genetic theories, psychoanalytic theory, developmental theories, theories relating to family therapy or family sociology, and theories derived from the expanding knowledge in gerontology.

Evolutionary-genetic theories stress the biological aspects of grandparenthood. The Evolutionary-Biology Theory (Kornhaber 1996; Turke 1988), for instance, highlights the association between the average age at which men and women become grandfathers and grandmothers and their entrance into the infertile stage, biologically speaking, in their lives. It holds that when individuals, especially women, no longer have the biological ability to give birth, they are more available to provide assistance and support to their children and grandchildren, who represent their biological continuity. This theory also explains the more meaningful relationship established between maternal grandparents and their grandchildren as compared to that of paternal grandparents, arguing that maternal grandparents know for certain that the grandchildren represent their biological continuity and are therefore more highly motivated to invest in their lives (Smith 1991). Another theory in this category is the Genetic Similarity Theory, which maintains that the quality of the grandparent-grandchild relationship is a function of the similarity between them. In support of this notion, Leek and Smith (1991) found that similarity in personality between grandparents and grandchildren was associated with higher involvement, investment, and assistance on the part of the grandparents in the grandchildren's care.

Another theoretical approach to grandparenthood derives from *psychoanalysis*. Scholars adopting this perspective pioneered the application of concepts such as "Oedipal conflict" and "transference" to the role grandparents play in the psychological development of their grandchildren. Thus, for example, Strauss (1943) explained how the child's castration anxiety toward his father could be transferred to the grandfather. Using the same reasoning, Battistelli and Farneti (1991) describe the grandparents as a substitute for the parents in assisting adolescent grandchildren through the process of separation/individuation. Integrating traditional psychoanalytic thinking and the sociodemographic features of modern society, Robinson (1989) notes that most individuals whose offspring have grown up and left home expect to become grandparents. For those who were busy with their careers when they were parents, grandparenthood may be an opportunity to re-experience child rearing. In addition, their grandchildren's struggle with developmental conflicts (such as the Oedipal conflict) may provide a chance for them to reprocess unresolved developmental conflicts from the past. Nonetheless, Robinson (1989) claims that some grandparents do not wish to invest in the grandparent role or can not do so for a variety of reasons. They may still have an active career, may live at a geographical distance from their grandchildren, or may have aging parents who depend on them. In some cases, unresolved conflicts with their children may hinder their involvement with the grandchildren.

A further category of theoretical approaches to grandparenthood are *developmental theories*. The most relevant one was devised by Erikson (1963), who describes eight developmental stages in the life span. The final stage, which occurs in late adulthood, centers around the developmental conflict between ego integrity and despair. According to this theory, the transition to grandparenthood symbolizes the loss of fertility and the start of the last phase of life. In this period, people review their lives, summing up their achievements and recognizing the goals they have not achieved. Grandparenthood can also promote acceptance of the cycle of life, whereby the birth of a new generation brings the older generation closer to inevitable death. Erikson et al. (1986) argue that one way to successfully resolve the conflict at this stage of life is by caring for grandchildren. The authors claim that in contrast to the fertility embedded in previous stages, which enables the individual to create and nurture children, the final stage is characterized by helping to shape the next generation and enhancing the Grand Generativity, or intergenerational continuity. In an extension of his theory written late in his life, Erikson (1982) stated that old age includes integration of all previous developmental stages, thus reflecting both change and continuity.

A more recent theoretical framework is *life span developmental psychology*, which evolved out of gerontology. This approach integrates concepts from developmental psychology and family sociology (Baltes et al. 1980), stressing the continuity of developmental processes throughout the life span and the way in which they are influenced by biological, psychological, and normative social factors. Moreover, it relates to the timing of life transitions in light of social expectations and historical events in the individual's life span (Shmotkin 2003). Bengston (1987), for example, differentiates between the concepts of "generation" and "cohort," with the former referring to the familial relationship between parents and their children and the latter to the historical and social events that shape the role of a certain age group. These terms are used to examine the direct influences (family relations) and indirect influences (historical and social events) of the grandparents' generation on that of the grandchildren (Smith 2002). From this perspective, grandparents are seen to constitute a moderating factor in family circumstances such as divorce and other stressful and disruptive family events or social contexts such as wars (Smith 2002; Woodbridge et al. 2011).

The development of *family theories* shone the spotlight on the role that grandparents, as extended family, may play in family functioning. The Family Systems Theory, a leader in this category, holds that family members form a system in which each member is in an interaction with all the others. Thus, any change in one family member upsets the balance of the whole system, which then struggles to regain a state of balance (Cox and Paley 1997; Walsh and McGraw 1996). Changes can be normative, such as the transition to parenthood or grandparenthood, or non-normative, such as divorce or illness. “Healthy” families are said to be characterized by boundaries that protect the members, but are flexible enough to allow them to adapt to change. Such families respect the unique characteristics of each member, as well as the unique style of the family as a whole (Minuchin 1974). Acknowledging the important role grandparents play in the healthy functioning of the family system, therapists began to invite them to participate in family interventions (Haley 1976; Minuchin et al. 1967). One of the problems encountered in the course of therapy is the way families build triple relationships to bypass conflicts, anxieties, or inconvenience, a phenomenon termed the “detouring triangle” (Miller and Sandberg 1998). For example, grandparents in dispute with their offspring may use their grandchildren to transmit messages to their parents or obtain information about them. A unique kind of family intervention is the “Filial/Family Play Therapy (FFPT) grandparent training model”. This intervention is conducted among custodial grandparents and aimed at fostering healthy parent-child relationships through training and supervising grandparents in the basic methodology of child-centered play therapy, while providing them with the emotional support they need. Grandparents conduct weekly play therapy-type sessions with their grandchild; learning to convey acceptance, empathy, and encouragement, as well as master the skills of effective limit setting (Bratton et al. 2006).

A final category in the discourse on grandparenthood are *theories of aging*. In contrast to the situation in traditional societies, grandparents in the modern world no longer enjoy the status of “elders” (Sangree 1992; Thomas et al. 2000), and may not even be biologically old. Research in gerontology relates, among other things, to age stereotypes regarding grandparents, even when the individual is relatively young. Moreover, the literature reveals that most people will continue to serve as grandparents during their young-old, middle-old, and old-old years, which necessitates dealing with the multigenerational effects of both the negative consequences of aging, such as dementia (Creasey et al. 1989), and the more positive consequences, such as a mature moral perception and greater wisdom (Clayton and Birren 1980).

Contemporary research tends to view grandparenthood as a construct influenced by multiple factors. The multidimensional Intergenerational Solidarity Model (Bengston and Mangen 1988) depicts the complex relationships between parents and their children and between grandparents and their grandchildren, relating to family habitation, intergenerational relationship patterns, the quality of intergenerational relations, the level of similarity between family members in regard to values, attitudes, and beliefs, perceptions of support and mutuality in providing support, and the extent of agreement on commitment to fulfill family roles. All these elements impact relations in the family system, with parents being obliged to the intergenerational norms more than any other generation, as they are committed both to their aging parents and to the children who are still dependent on them (Hirdes and Strain 1995). Recognition of the importance of intergenerational relations has led to an increase in recent years of research conducted from a three-generational perspective (e.g., Werner et al. 2005), an issue discussed extensively below in the section on the grandparent-grandchild relationship.

The various approaches to the subject of grandparenthood also project on how the role of the grandparent is perceived and defined.

1.3 Definition of the Grandparent Role

The dictionary defines "grandparent" as the parent of a child's father or mother. Restricting the definition to attributional-biological status, however, gives no hint of the complexity of the role of this family member, which is, in fact, defined by a wide range of psychological, social, and perceptional/attitudinal features of the individual and their society (Clavan 1978). Clavan (1978) highlights this complexity by defining grandparenthood as a "roleless role", that is, a role without any obligations or rights like that of parent. This section reviews the ways this role has been defined in the empirical literature over the years, from the first studies that focused mainly on the role dimensions or the different types of grandparents, to a recent extensive study which merged these dimensions into an integrative model.

In a pioneering study, Neugarten and Weinstein (1964) defined five grandparenting styles:

1. **Formal**. A strict division of roles between the parents and grandparents is maintained. While the grandparents show an interest in their grandchildren, they are not involved in child rearing.
2. **Fun seeker**. The grandparents play with the child and both sides derive pleasure from the interactions.
3. **Surrogate**. The grandparents assume the parental role of caregivers and child rearing because parents are absent or work long hours.

Although Neugarten and Weinstein (1964) related to grandmothers who care for their grandchildren while their mothers are at work, over the years this category has been extended to include grandparents who take over responsibility for the children because the parents can not perform this function due to problems such as addiction, couple conflicts, mental disease, poverty, or incarceration (Waldrop and Weber 2001). In such circumstances, grandparents become the main caregivers and are termed "parental grandparents", In other cases they may serve as "near-parental grandparents", caring for their grandchildren while the parents are at work or raising the children together with the parents in the same household (Lumpkin 2008).

Lumpkin (2008) notes that the number of American studies which deal with surrogate grandparents is considerably higher than those dealing with "regular" grandparents, and quotes Census Bureau statistics showing that in 2000, 2.5 million grandparents in the US were raising their grandchildren, 38 % of them for a period of over 5 years. This arrangement is most common among grandmothers and in African American and Hispanic families (Szinovacz 1998). Surrogate grandparents have been shown to experience more financial problems (Bullock 2004), health problems (Hughes et al. 2007), depression (Musil and Ahmad 2002), and social isolation (Bullock 2004). When such difficulties are joined by behavioral problems on the part of the grandchild, the level of stress with which surrogate grandparents have to cope is intensified (Harrison et al. 2000).

Nevertheless, most grandparents do not take over the parental role. Many, however, still have to deal with their children's expectation that they will help with raising the grandchildren so that they can continue to study and develop professionally (Ben Shlomo and Taubman – Ben-Ari 2012). Thus, in many ways, they may experience stress levels similar to those of surrogate grandparents (Ben Shlomo 2014).

4. **Reservoir of family wisdom**. The grandparents are the autohrity in the family, taking the responsibility to pass the family legacy to future generations.

Neugarten and Weinstein (1964) attributed this style mainly to grandfathers who occupy a position of authority in the family. In studies conducted in later years, it was extended to grandmothers as well. It features, for example, in Kivnick's (1982) discussion of grandparenthood as an opportunity to reexperience one's personal past. Tinsley and Parke (1984) refer to it as the function of "family historian" responsible for passing on the family legacy, and Bengston (1985) speaks of the social construction of biography. According to Bengston (1985), grandparents inject unique meanings into their grandchildren's present through integration with their own past. The current theoretical discourse tends to relate to grandparents in the context of the extended family system, suggesting a holistic approach whereby the transmission of values and family legacy is a process that takes place in the whole family system and involves both parents and grandparents (Mueller and Elder 2003).

5. **Distant figure**. The grandparents have fleeting contact with their grandchildren, remaining remote from their lives and only infrequently displaying affection.

The styles defined by Neugarten and Weinstein (1964) relate to different levels of grandparents' involvement in the lives of their grandchildren. Whereas the authors offered only a description of the styles, other researchers have focused on factors which may lead to the adoption of one or another. Kornhaber (1996), for instance, claims that every problem in family functioning should also be examined from the perspective of the grandparents' functioning. Based on interviews with 300 couples of grandmothers and grandfathers, he points to three involvement disorders. The first is identity disorder, characterized by the lack of involvement in the life of the grandchild. According to the author, this stems from a personality disorder such as narcissism. The second is activity disorder, in which grandparents treat their grandchildren as if they were their parents, or are unable to adapt to the changing developmental needs of the child. The third malfunction is communication disorder, reflected in forgetting important family events, being late for visits with the grandchild, or lack of communication.

In addition to conceptualizing the five grandparental styles, Neugarten and Weinstein (1964) also dealt with five meanings grandparents attach to their role, viewing grandparenthood as: a source of biological renewal and continuity; a resource promoting satisfaction and self-fulfillment; an opportunity to provide guidance and direction in regard to family values; a chance to offer their grandchildren emotional support; or a meaningless role.

Other studies have related to the symbolic meaning of the grandparent role, such as intergenerational continuity (Hurme 1991; Kahana and Kahana 1971), or intergenerational moderation (Bengston 1985). Some studies have found that the role itself may contribute to a sense of meaning in life (Kivnick 1982), while others indicate that role satisfaction is an important aspect for a sense of meaning (Hurme 1991). Recent years have witnessed the emergence and development of positive psychology, resulting in a growing body of literature examining grandparenthood as an opportunity for personal development and growth (e.g., Taubman – Ben-Ari et al. 2012a, b), as well as an opportunity to enhance the meaning in life of the older generation (Taubman – Ben-Ari et al. 2012a).

This review of existing literature indicates the multifaceted experience of grandparenthood on the one hand, and the lack of a systematic theoretical framework for the analysis of accumulating knowledge on the other. Szinovacz (1998) maintains that one of the problems with research on grandparents is that it is based largely on case studies or relatively small and non-representative samples, and does not have a clear theoretical footing. An attempt to create such a framework was undertaken by a group of Israeli researchers (Findler et al. 2013), who constructed a comprehensive model along with a set of self-report inventories designed to examine the Multidimensional Experience of Grandparenthood (MEG). The model consists of four dimensions based on Hurme's (1991) conceptualization of grandparenthood: the *cognitive* dimension, referring to perceptions of the rights and obligations of grandparents, and conceptualized in the model as the way in which grandparents perceive their role; the *behavioral* dimension, relating to the activities involved in the role, and conceptualized as patterns of instrumental, financial, and emotional support; the *emotional* dimension, conceptualized as role satisfaction and the affects aroused by the role; and the *symbolic* dimension, which relates to a sense of continuity and personal satisfaction and is conceptualized in the model as the representative value attributed to the role. A basic assumption of the model is that the four dimensions are interrelated and are affected by a diversity of factors, including grandparents' personal characteristics and features of the family.

The study conducted by Findler et al. (2013) on a sample of 313 Israeli grandparents provided strong evidence for the value of distinguishing among the different domains of grandparenthood, as well as for the internal reliability and validity of the MEG and its ability to explain variations in the experience of grandparenthood. The results confirmed the four dimensions of grandparenthood proposed by Hurme (1991). Moreover, they indicated further complexity within each of the dimensions, and showed that positive and negative features of the experience of grandparenthood may exist side by side. More specifically, it was found that the cognitive dimension contains two contrasting factors which relate to commitment to the role of grandparenthood: the motivation to invest time and effort and the perceived personal cost in terms of priorities, time, and money. The affective dimension was also shown to consist of two conflicting factors: positive feelings of joy, accomplishment, and pride and negative feelings of anger, guilt, or disappointment. The behavioral dimension was found to contain three significant factors: emotional support, expressed in kissing, hugging, and encouraging the grandchildren; contribution to upbringing, reflected in shared activities that enrich the grandchildren or contribute to their development, such as storytelling or arts and crafts projects; and instrumental support, such as babysitting, bathing the grandchildren, or cooking for them. Four significant factors were found in the symbolic dimension: meaning, that is, the sense that grandparenthood is a uniquely enriching and challenging experience; compensation for parenthood, or the sense that grandparenthood is more rewarding and satisfying than parenthood; continuity, representing the intergenerational bond and the link between past and future; and burden, the perception of grandparenthood as burdensome and inconvenient.

This multidimensional approach to the analysis of the grandparent role makes it possible to relate to a variety of aspects and offers insights into the complexity of this stage in the life of the older individual, an understanding that appears to have been lacking in previous years, at least in the empirical literature. It also opens a vast array of options for exploring grandparenthood and its diverse features and relating them to other aspects of human life, including sociodemographic variables, personality, social support systems, and the socio-cultural environment.

1.4 The Relationship Between Grandparents and Grandchildren

As noted above, early studies of the grandparent-grandchild relationship tended to ignore the impact of other members of the family, such as the parents, the other set of grandparents, or additional grandchildren, as well as unique features of the grandparents and grandchildren themselves (King et al. 1998). A change in this approach has been seen in recent years with the rise of the family system theory (Cox and Paley 1997; Klein and White 1996), which, as noted above, regards each family member not only as an individual, but also as part of the family unit, both influencing and being influenced by it. According to this approach, family members are interconnected, maintaining material, emotional, and symbolic relationships with each other while at the same time interacting with their physical and social environment. Thus, the contemporary literature views the relationship between grandparents and grandchildren as part of the wider web of relations in the family system.

The theoretical perspective of exchange relations sheds light on several elements which may contribute to the grandparent-grandchild relationship. These include grandparents' personal characteristics, their relations with their children (the child's parents), the living arrangement and geographical proximity or distance, and socio cultural norms.

In regard to personal characteristics, age appears to be particularly relevant, with findings indicating that younger grandparents maintain a closer relationship with their grandchildren (Thomas 1989). In a study of college students, for example, Kennedy (1991) found that those with younger grandparents (aged 50–60) associated grandparents with love, intimacy and shared activities, while among those whose grandparents were older (aged 75 and over), the primary association was with providing care for the older generation. Indeed, serious health problems, which are more likely to appear in later life, may mitigate the quality of the intergenerational relationship (Creasey et al. 1989).

Grandparent's age has also been examined in relation to grandchild's age. King et al. (1998) claim that the relationship is dynamic and changes over time. A grandmother in her 50s and her two-year-old grandson will engage in different activities than a 75-year-old grandmother and her 22-year-old grandson. Older grandparents tend to offer their older grandchildren advice and support, while younger intergenerational relationships are characterized primarily by fun activities and babysitting.

Gender and lineage (maternal or paternal) have also been found to be related to the nature of the relationship between grandparents and their grandchildren. Most studies report that grandmothers are more involved than grandfathers in their grandchildren's lives (e.g., Roberto and Stroes 1992). Recent studies, however, indicate that grandfathers express a willingness to play a more meaningful part in the life of their grandchildren than reflected in the level of their actual involvement (e.g., Waldrop et al. 1999). Such findings suggest that a new pattern of grandparenthood may be evolving in modern society, although this possibility has yet to be thoroughly explored.

In regard to lineage, research indicates that maternal grandparents are more involved in the care of their grandchildren than paternal grandparents (Wheelock and Jones 2002). Smith (1991) suggests that these findings are a reflection of the close relationship which typically exists between mothers and daughters, and may also be enhanced by social expectations.

Another personal characteristic which may impact the grandparent-grandchild relationship is the existence of additional grandchildren in the family. One study has found that the greater the number of grandchildren, the more difficult it is for grandparents to establish a close relationship with each one separately (King and Elder 1995). Furthermore, Fingerman (1998) found that the particular traits of each of the grandchildren may engender a preference for one over the others. Thus, the quality of the grandparent-grandchild relationship may also be associated with the extent to which a grandchild's individual characteristics cause the grandparent to feel special affection for him or her.

In regard to personality traits Mansson (2015), a communication scholar, indicates that grandchildren have several expectations about their grandparents' attributes and behaviors, such as being caring, comforting, family-oriented, generous, kind, loving, supportive, trustworthy and understanding.

In addition, empirical findings indicate that the parents make a significant contribution to the grandparent-grandchild relationship. They can either promote the connection or go so far as to actually sabotage its existence (King and Elder 1995).

Living arrangements and geographical proximity are also of great importance. A shared household, in which the three generations live together, creates closer intergenerational relationships, encouraging grandparents to become meaningful figures in their grandchildren's lives (King and Elder 1995). Such an arrangement is more common in rural than in urban areas. When parents and grandparents live apart, the geographical distance becomes significant (Boon and Brussoni 1996; Hodgson 1992). In fact, Kivett (1991) found that in 93 % of the cases in which a close relationship was reported between grandparents and grandchildren, they lived in close proximity to one another.

Finally, the cultural context also plays an important role in shaping the grandparent-grandchild relationship. In China, where triadic familial habitation is the norm, there is greater proximity between grandparents and grandchildren (Shu 1999). In Kenya and Nigeria, grandparents are revered as the tribal elders, with obvious implications for their relations with their grandchildren (Sangree 1992); in Arab cultures, which are characterized by collectivist values, grandparents are looked up to as individuals from whose experience and wisdom one can learn (Dwairy 2002); in African American families in the US, maternal grandmothers enjoy a special status and are a major source of support for their grandchildren, among other things because of the large number of single-parent families in which grandmothers serve as custodial caretakers for their grandchildren (Borenstein 2002). It is important to note, however, that most of the research on grandparenthood has been conducted in the United States and other western societies, making it difficult to determine whether the findings can be applied to non-western cultures. In this respect, research performed in Israel is of particular value. While Israel resembles other western cultures, it also displays features more commonly found in traditional, conservative societies, such as close family ties.

1.5 The Emotional Experience of Grandparenthood

To date, most information about the emotional reaction to grandparenthood comes from popular literature. In *The Birth of a Grandmother* (Harari 2006), for example, the author, a social psychologist, presents the stories of new grandmothers who meet with her once a week in order to verbalize and share their feelings and thoughts following this life transition. For one woman, it arouses memories of her relationship with her own grandmother:

Whenever I hear the word grandma, I immediately see my grandmother. She was a real grandmother, there was a lot of love between us. It was a different love from the one I felt from my mother. It was also a completely different relationship. In my relationship with my grandmother, there was nothing intimidating. Grandma was a grandmother not a mother (Harari 2006, p. 55).

For another woman, who never knew her grandmother, the birth of a grandchild made her keenly aware of what she had missed out on:

Only now, suddenly, when I am a grandmother, my heart aches to think that no grandmother ever held me like that in her arms. It was never as concrete as right now, and I really pity myself and I'm saddened to think about what I was lacking. Only now when I hug my grandson, hold him, bring him close to my heart, I say, what a terrible thing (Harari 2006, p. 59).

These descriptions illustrate the strong emotions aroused by grandparenthood and the variations in the experience, a subject that has thus far received scant research attention.

1.6 The Impact of Changing Family Models on Grandparenthood

New family models are becoming increasingly common in modern society. Two such models appear to be particularly salient to the issue of grandparenthood: single-parent families resulting from separation or divorce; and families of same-sex couples.

The growth in divorce rates in Britain and the United States (Rodgers and Pryor 1998) has spawned considerable research into the effects of divorce on the parent-child relationship. A much smaller body of literature deals with the relationship between the children and their grandparents (Borenstein 2002). These studies indicate that when grandparent-parent relations remain good, grandparents may provide support, both financial and emotional, as well as a sense of stability (Kennedy and Kennedy 1993; Kivett 1991; Uhlenberg and Cheuk 2010). Furthermore, they may serve as a moderating factor for the increased stress in the family that derives from the divorce (Henderson et al. 2009; Yorgason and Gustafson 2014). This contribution is even stronger when the grandparents' physical health is good and when they live in close proximity to their grandchildren (Borenstein 2002). However, a problematic relationship with the custodial parent may interfere with the quality of the grandparent-grandchild relationship (Kruk 1995), which often means that paternal grandparents are at greater risk of an impaired relationship with their grandchildren following separation or divorce (Kruk and Hall 1995).

Another growing phenomenon in modern western society is same-sex families. The few studies that have been conducted on this population relate mainly to the parents and to the complex situations arising from the new technologies available, such as a child conceived from the sperm of one of the partners and a donor egg which is then implanted into the womb of a surrogate mother. To the best of our knowledge, only two studies have dealt with the role of the grandparents in same-sex families, both relating to female couples. The first (Patterson et al. 1998) interviewed 37 lesbian mothers of children aged 4–9, and found that most of the children met monthly with their grandparents. Such children were shown to have fewer behavioral problems than those who did not have regular contact with their grandparents. Furthermore, the grandchildren's relationship with their biological grandparents was stronger and more meaningful than with their non-biological grandparents. The second study (Fulcher et al. 2005) compared the young children of lesbian and heterosexual mothers, and found similar contact with the grandparents in both groups. Here, too, the relationship with the biological grandparents was shown to be closer among all the children.

Although nothing could be found in the professional literature concerning the emotional experience of grandparents in these two family models, numerous Internet sites are aimed specifically at this sector. Here they can find not only technical and/or legal information, but also sources offering social and emotional support, indicating the existence of unique issues with which grandparents are confronted as a result of the new families in modern society.

1.7 Grandparenthood in Theory and Research: An Overview

Our review of the theory and research on grandparenthood reveals the changes that have taken place over the years. The theoretical approach has shifted its focus, moving from intrapersonal processes, as in the psychoanalytic theory, through the perception of grandparenting as a developmental task, as in Erikson's developmental theory (1982), to an intergenerational model which centers around interactions among all members of the family system. This change is also reflected in the definition of the grandparent role. Whereas the pioneering study by Neugarten and Weinstein (1964) defined different types of grandparents based on the degree of their involvement in their grandchild's life, contemporary research aims at a multidimensional examination of grandparenthood (e.g., Findler et al. 2013), relating to features of the family system as a whole, such as prolonged longevity and changes in fertility patterns, characteristics of the individuals in the system, including age, gender, lineage, and education, and environmental factors which determine the context in which the family functions, such as culture, place of residence, and social and familial stressors. As noted above, this broad approach indicates the complexity and diversity of the grandparenting experience, as well as the lack of a firm theoretical foundation for its study.

Although recent years have witnessed a considerable growth in research devoted to grandparents, many aspects have yet to be examined. One reason may be the salience of old age and proximity of death which are associated with the transition to grandparenthood and with grandparenting itself (Kahana and Kahana 1971). This may indeed have been the reality in the past, when life expectancy was lower and people became grandparents close to the end of life (Tinsley and Parke 1984). However, at a time when the transition to grandparenthood generally takes place in middle age (Smith 2002), the associations with old age and death are mainly symbolic (Gauthier 2002). Nevertheless, it is possible that such stereotypes continue to arouse anxiety, even among researchers, discouraging them from dealing with the subject of grandparenthood. In addition, as we have shown, existing research relates to various aspects of grandparenting, but does not give sufficient weight to the affective experience of being a grandfather or grandmother. Additional studies, most of them presumably qualitative, are needed to broaden our understanding of this issue. The approach of positive psychology, which has gained momentum in recent decades, may provide a context in which to examine the ability of grandparents to thrive and grow as a result of their role, even in challenging circumstances such as the security situation in Israel or the shaky financial situation in the US and Europe.

Another interesting avenue of research is the effect of modern family. One question worth investigating is whether the media today portrays a more realistic image of grandparents or whether it preserves the traditional stereotype. Two studies published in 2010 (Sciplino et al. 2010) show a very stereotypical media representations of grandparents in Europe. Study 1 explores how grandparents are depicted in children's books: 149 images (87 grandmothers, 62 grandfathers) were obtained from children's picture books in Britain, Italy, and Greece. Results of content analysis point that seventy percent of grandfathers and 59 % of grandmothers have gray/white hair. More than 50 % of grandparents are in sedentary physical activities: sitting, standing, lying in bed, and reading. Study 2 investigates whether the apparent age of grandparents in children's books differs by gender, nationality, or year of book publication in Britain, Italy, Greece, Finland, and Poland. Twelve adults in Britain and Italy and 10 adults in Finland estimated the age of each grandparent figure (from 40–44 years old to 90+). In every country, grandfathers were rated as significantly older than grandmothers. Grandparents are significantly older in Greek books than in British books and are significantly older in Polish books than in Finnish books. In Britain, Italy, Greece, and Finland, grandparents in children's books are older than the estimated average age of grandparents with young grandchildren. Developments in the media have also opened new channels that may impact grandparents in general and grandparent media representation in particular. These developments offering different options for communication between grandparents and their grandchildren than in the past. Social networks, such as Facebook and Twitter, enable grandparents to share their grandchildren's experiences without the mediation of the parents; technologies such as Skype provide for free transatlantic conversations, including video calls, allowing grandparents to follow their grandchildren's growth even from a distance.

Such possibilities raise questions regarding the importance of geographical distance between grandparents and grandchildren as a factor in their relationship, as well as ethical questions regarding to grandparents' ability to obtain information about their grandchildren and bypass the parents. Indeed, given the changes both in society and in technology, the future mode of grandparent-grandchild relationship may be very different than what we are accustomed to.

In the coming years, research will also have to develop reliable instruments to measure the complex family and environmental processes that play a part in grandparenthood (for example, how perceived career stress is related to the grandparent role). Statistical methods suitable for such measurements will have to be devised as well.

Finally, accumulating empirical knowledge poses new challenges for clinical practice. It suggests the need to develop interventions specially designed for grandparents that address both personal concerns and intergenerational dynamics.

References

Baltes, P. B., Reese, H. W., & Lipsitt, L. P. (1980). Life–span developmental psychology. *Annual Review of Psychology, 31*, 65–100.

Barranti, C. C. R. (1985). The grandparent—grandchild relationship: Family resource in an era of voluntary bond. *Family Relations, 34*, 343–352.

Battistelli, P., & Farneti, A. (1991). Grandchildren's images of their grandparents: A psychodynamic perspective. In P. K. Smith (Ed.), *The psychology of grandparenthood: An international perspective* (pp. 143–156). London: Routledge.

Ben Shlomo, S. (2014). What makes first time grandparents more satisfied with life? *Stress & Health, 30*, 23–33.

Ben Shlomo, S., & Taubman – Ben-Ari, O. (2012). New grandparents mental health: The protective role of optimism, self-mastery and social support. *Journal of Family Social Work, 15*, 254–271.

Bengston, V. L. (1985). Diversity and symbolism in grandparental roles. In V. L. Bengston & J. F. Robertson (Eds.), *Grandparenthood* (pp. 11–25). Beverly Hills, CA: Sage.

Bengston, V. L. (1987). Parenting, grandparenting and life intergenerational continuity. In J. B. Lancaster, J. Altmann, A. S. Rossi, & L. R. Sherrod (Eds.), *Parenting across the life span: Biosocial dimensions* (pp. 435–456). New York, NY: Aldine de Gruyter.

Bengston, V. L., & Mangen, D. J. (1988). Family intergenerational solidarity revised. In D. J. Mangen, V. L. Bengston, & P. H. Landry (Eds.), *Measurement of intergenerational relations* (pp. 222–238). Beverly Hills, CA: Sage.

Boon, S. D., & Brussoni, M. J. (1996). Young adults' relationships with their closest grandparents: Examining emotional closeness. *Journal of Social Behavior and Personality, 11*, 439–458.

Borenstein, M. H. (2002). *Handbook of parenting: Being and becoming a parent*. Mahwah, NJ: Erlbaum.

Bratton, S., Ray, D., & Moffit, K. (2006). Fillial/Family play therapy: An intervention for custodial grandparents and their grandchildren. *Educational Gerontology, 24*, 391–406.

Bullock, K. (2004). The changing role of grandparents in rural families: The results of exploratory study in southeastern North Carolina. *Families in Society, 85*, 45–54.

Clavan, S. (1978). The impact of social class and social trends on the role of the grandparent. *The Family Coordinator, 27*, 351–357.

Clayton, V. P., & Birren, J. E. (1980). The development of wisdom across the life span: A reexamination of an ancient topic. *Life-span development and behavior, 3*, 103–135.

Cox, M. J., & Paley, B. (1997). Families as systems. *Annual Review of Psychology, 48*, 243–267.

Creasey, G. L., Myers, B. J., Epperson, M. J., & Taylor, J. (1989). Grandchildren of grandparents with Alzheimer's disease: Perceptions of grandparent, family environment, and the elderly. *Merrill-Palmer Quarterly, 35*, 227–237.

Dwairy, M. (2002). Foundations of a psycho-social dynamic personality theory of collective people. *Clinical Psychology Review, 22*, 343–360.

Erikson, E. H. (1963). *Childhood and society* (2nd ed.). New York, NY: Norton.

Erikson, E. H. (1982). *The life cycle completed: A review*. New York, NY: Norton.

Erikson, E. H., Erikson, J. M., & Kivnick, H. Q. (1986). *Vital involvement in old age*. New York, NY: Norton.

Findler, L., Taubman - Ben-Ari, O., Nuttman-Shwartz, O., & Lazar, R. (2013). Construction and validation of the multidimensional experience of grandparenthood set of inventories (MEG). *Social Work Research, 37*, 237–253.

Fingerman, K. L. (1998). The good, the bad, and the worrisome: Emotional complexities in grandparents' experiences with individual grandchildren. *Family Relations, 47*, 403–414.

Fulcher, M., Sutfin, E. L., Chan, R. W., Scheib, J. E., & Patterson, C. J. (2005). Lesbian mothers and their children: Findings from the contemporary families study. In A. Omoto & H. Kurtzman (Eds.), *Recent research on sexual orientation, mental health, and substance abuse* (pp. 281–299). Washington, DC: American Psychological Association.

Gauthier, A. (2002). The role of grandparents. *Current Sociology, 50*, 295–307.

Haley, J. (1976). *Problem-solving therapy: New strategies for effective family therapy*. San Francisco, CA: Jossey-Bass.

Harari, A. (2006). *Birth of a grandmother [Holedet sabta]*. Babel (Hebrew): Tel Aviv.

Harrison, K. A., Richman, G. S., & Vittimberga, G. L. (2000). Parental stress in grandparents versus parents raising children with behavior problems. *Journal of Family Issues, 21*, 262–270.

Henderson, C. E., Hayslip, B., Sanders, L. M., & Louden, L. (2009). Grandmother–grandchild relationship quality predicts psychological adjustment among youth from divorced families. *Journal of Family Issues*, 1264–1245 *,30*

Hirdes, J. P., & Strain, L. A. (1995). The balance of exchange in instrumental support with network members outside the household. *Journal of Gerontology: Social Sciences, 50*, 134–142.

Hodgson, L. G. (1992). Adult grandchildren and their grandparents—The enduring bond. *International Journal of Aging and Human Development, 34*, 209–225.

Hughes, M. E., Waite, L. J., LaPierre, T. A., & Luo, Y. (2007). All in the family: The impact of caring for grandchildren on grandparents' health. *Journal of Gerontology B: Psychological & Social Sciences, 62*, 108–119.

Hurme, H. (1991). Dimensions of the grandparent role in Finland. In P. K. Smith (Ed.), *The Psychology of grandparenthood: An international perspective* (pp. 19–31). New York, NY: Routledge.

Johnson, C. L., & Troll, L. (1996). Family structure and the timing of transitions from 70 to 103 years of age. *Journal of Marriage and Family, 58*, 178–187.

Kahana, E., & Kahana, B. (1971). Theoretical and research perspectives on grandparenthood. *Aging & Human Development, 2*, 261–268.

Kennedy, G. E. (1991). Quality in grandparent/grandchild relationships. *International journal of aging & human development, 35*, 83–98.

Kennedy, G. E., & Kennedy, C. E. (1993). Grandparents: A special resource for children in stepfamilies. *Journal of Divorce & Remarriage, 19*, 45–68.

King, V., & Elder, G. H. (1995). American children view their grandparents: Linked lives across three rural generations. *Journal of Marriage & the Family, 57*, 165–178.

King, V., Russell, S. T., & Elder, G. H. (1998). Grandparenting in family systems: An ecological perspective. In M. Szinovacz (Ed.), *Handbook on grandparenthood* (pp. 53–69). Westport, CT: Greenwood Press.

Kivett, V. R. (1991). The grandparent–grandchild connection. *Marriage & Family Review, 16*, 267–290.

Kivnick, H. Q. (1982). *The meaning of grandparenthood*. Ann Arbor, MI: UMI Research Press.
Klein, D. M., & White, J. M. (1996). The systems framework. In J. M. White, D. M. Klein, & T. F. Martin (Eds.), *Family theories* (pp. 117–142). London: Sage Publications.
Kornhaber, A. (1996). *Contemporary grandparenting*. Thousand Oaks, CA: Sage.
Kruk, E. (1995). Grandparent-grandchild contact loss: Findings from a study of "Grandparent Rights" members. *Canadian Journal on Aging, 14*, 737–754.
Kruk, E., & Hall, B. (1995). The disengagement of paternal grandparents subsequent to divorce. *Journal of Divorce and Remarriage, 23*, 131–147.
Leek, M., & Smith, P. K. (1991). Cooperation and conflict in three–generation families. In P. K. Smith (Ed.), *The psychology of grandparenthood: An international perspective* (pp. 177–194). London: Routledge.
Lowenstein, A. (2010). Intergenerational relations in the aging family. In Y. Brick & A. Lowenstein (Eds.), *The elderly and the family* (pp. 629–640). Jerusalem: Eshel (Hebrew).
Lumpkin, J. R. (2008). Grandparents in a parental or near-parental role: Sources of stress and coping mechanisms. *Journal of Family Issues, 29*, 357–372.
Mansson, D. H. (2015). Developing the ideal grandparent scale: Initial validity and reliability tests. *Journal of Intergenerational Relationships, 13*, 207–226.
Miller, R. B., & Sandberg, J. G. (1998). Clinical intervention in intergenerational relations. In M. Szinovacz (Ed.), *Handbook on grandparenthood* (pp. 217–229). Westport, CT: Greenwood Press.
Minuchin, S. (1974). *Families and family therapy*. Cambridge, MA: Harvard University Press.
Minuchin, S., Montalvo, B., Guerney, B. G., Rosman, B. L., & Schumer, F. (1967). *Families of the slums*. New York: Basic Books.
Mueller, M. M., & Elder, G. H. (2003). Family contingencies across the generations: Grandparent-grandchild relationships in holistic perspective. *Journal of Marriage and Family, 65*, 404–417.
Musil, C. M., & Ahmad, M. (2002). Health of grandmothers: A comparison by caregiver status. *Journal of Aging and Health, 14*, 96–121.
Neugarten, B. L., & Weinstein, K. (1964). The changing American grandparent. *Journal of Marriage and the Family, 26*, 199–204.
Patterson, C., Hurt, S., & Mason, C. (1998). Families of the lesbian baby-boom: Children's contact with grandparents and other adults. *American Journal of Orthopsychiatry, 68*, 390–399.
Rappaport, E. A. (1958). The grandparent syndrome. *The Psychoanalytic Quarterly, 27*, 518–538.
Roberto, K. A., & Stroes, J. (1992). Grandchildren and grandparents: Roles, influences, and relationships. *International Journal of Aging and Human Development, 34*, 227–239.
Robinson, L. H. (1989). Grandparenting: Intergenerational love and hate. *The Journal of the American Academy of Psychoanalysis and Dynamic Psychiatry, 17*, 483–491.
Rodgers, B., & Pryor, J. (1998). *Divorce and separation: The outcomes for children*. York, UK: Joseph Rowntree Foundation.
Rossi, A. S., & Rossi, P. H. (1990). *Of human bonding: Parent–child relations across the life course*. New York, NY: Aldin de Gruyter.
Sangree, W. H. (1992). Grandparenthood and modernization: The changing status of male and female elders in Tiriki, Kenya, and Irigwe, Nigeria. *Journal of Cross Cultural Gerontology, 7*, 331–361.
Sciplino, C., Smith, P., Hurme, H., Busek, M., & Backvik, P. (2010). Representations of grandparents in children's books in Britain, Italy, Greece, Finland, and Poland. *Journal of Intergenerational Relationships, 8*, 298–316.
Shmotkin, D. (2003). Psychological theories of aging. In A. Rosin (Ed.), *Aging and gerontology in Israel* (pp. 345–383). Jerusalem: JDC-Eshel (Hebrew).
Shu, S. (1999). *Grandparents, parents and children: A study of three generation family structure and intergenerational relationships in contemporary China*. London: Goldsmiths College, University of London.

Silverstein, M., & Long, J. (1998). Trajectories of grandparents' perceived solidarity with adult grandchildren: A growth curve analysis over 23 years. *Journal of Marriage and the Family, 60*, 912–923.

Smith, M. S. (1991). An evolutionary perspective on grandparent–grandchild relationships. In P. K. Smith (Ed.), *The psychology of grandparenthood: An international perspective* (pp. 157–176). London: Routledge.

Smith, P. K. (2002). Grandparenthood. In M. H. Borenstein (Ed.), *Handbook of parenting* (Vol. 3, pp. 89–112)., Being and becoming a parent Hillsdale, NJ: Lawrence Erlbaum Associates.

Strauss, C. A. (1943). Grandma made Johnny delinquent. *American Journal of Orthopsychiatry, 13*, 343–347.

Szinovacz, M. E. (1998). Grandparents today: A demographic profile. *The Gerontologist, 38*, 37–52.

Taubman – Ben-Ari, O., Ben Shlomo, S., & Findler, L. (2012a). Personal growth and meaning in life among first-time mothers and grandmothers. *Journal of Happiness Studies, 13*, 801–820.

Taubman – Ben-Ari, O., Findler, L., & Ben Shlomo, S. (2012b). Personal growth and the transition to grandfatherhood. *The International Journal of Aging and Human Development, 74*, 265–285.

Thomas, J. L. (1989). Gender and grandparenthood. *International Journal of Aging and Human Development, 29*, 269–282.

Thomas, J. L., Sperry, L., & Yarbrough, M. S. (2000). Grandparents as parents, research, findings and policy recommendations. *Child Psychiatry and Human Development, 31*, 3–22.

Tinsley, B. J., & Parke, R. D. (1984). Grandparents as support and socialization agents. In M. Lewis (Ed.), *Beyond the dyad* (pp. 161–194). New York, NY: Plenum.

Troll, L. E. (1985). The contingencies of grandparenting. In V. L. Bengston & J. F. Robertson (Eds.), *Grandparenthood* (pp. 135–149). Beverly Hills, CA: Sage.

Turke, P. W. (1988). Helpers at the nest: Childcare networks on Ifaluk. In L. Betzig, M. Borgerhoff Mulder & P. Turke (Eds.), *Human reproductive behavior: A Darwinian perspective* (pp. 173–188). Cambridge, UK: Cambridge University Press.

Uhlenberg, P., & Cheuk, M. (2010). The significance of grandparents to grandchildren: An international perspective. In D. Dannefer & C. Phillipson (Eds.), *The SAGE handbook of social gerontology* (pp. 447–458). London, England: SAGE Publications Ltd.

Vollmer, H. (1937). The grandmother: A problem in child rearing. *American Journal of Orthopsychiatry, 7*, 378–382.

Waldrop, D. P., & Weber, J. A. (2001). From grandparent to caregiver: The stress and satisfaction of raising grandchildren. *Families in Society, 82*, 461–473.

Waldrop, D. P., Weber, J. A., Herald, S. L., Pruett, J., Cooper, K., & Juozapavicius, K. (1999). Wisdom and life experience: How grandfathers mentor their grandchildren. *Journal of Aging and Identity, 4*, 33–45.

Walsh, W. M., & McGraw, J. A. (1996). *Essentials of family therapy: A therapist's guide to eight approaches*. Denver, CO: Love Publishing Company.

Werner, P., Buchbinder, E., Lowenstein, A., & Livni, T. (2005). Mediation across generations: A tri-generational perspective. *Journal of Aging Studies, 19*, 489–502.

Wheelock, J., & Jones, K. (2002). 'Grandparents are the next best thing': Informal childcare for working parents in urban Britain. *Journal of Social Policy, 31*, 441–463.

Woodbridge, S., Buys, L., & Miller, E. (2011). "My grandchild has a disability": Impact on grandparenting identity, roles and relationships. *Journal of Aging Studies, 25*, 355–365.

Yorgason, J. B., & Gustafson, K. B. (2014). Linking grandparent involvement with the development of pro social behavior in adolescents. In L. M. Padilla-Walker & G. Carlo. (Eds.), *Prosocial development: A multidimensional approach* (pp. 201–220). New-York, NY: Oxford University Press.

Chapter 2
Becoming a Grandparent—On Transitions and Transformations

Adi Noy and Orit Taubman – Ben-Ari

Abstract The transition to grandparenthood brings with it a shift in status, roles, and identities, and is perceived by grandparents themselves as one of the most meaningful and emotional events in their lives. Nevertheless, it has only recently become the subject of comprehensive research. This chapter offers a wide view of grandparenthood from the perspective of the life cycle and other transitions, surveying various factors that shape the experience of the role, including age, gender, lineage, and frequency of meetings with the grandchild. The chapter also focuses on grandparents' psychological well-being and the process of personal growth, a positive psychological change that includes changes in self-perception, interpersonal relationships, and priorities, and may be triggered by becoming a grandparent.

Keywords Grandparenthood · Grandparents · Grandchildren · Life transition · Life cycle · Well-being · Personal growth · Positive psychology

> *Look, the enjoyment is remarkable. It did something incredible [to me] from many angles, emotionally and...essentially emotionally. It opens channels that... it isn't quite clear how it works. I think that there's even something hormonal involved, really, the body goes through something, not only the emotions. Something happens that's extremely powerful* (Grandmother)
>
> *I feel more complete, I feel I've accomplished the most meaningful mission there is in life* (Grandmother).

The transition to grandparenthood is one of the most significant and exciting events in adult life, and leads to changes in the individual, the family, and intrafamily relations. However, contrary to the wealth of research into other life events during adulthood, particularly the transition to parenthood (e.g., Cowan et al. 1985; Glade et al. 2005; Keizer and Schenk 2012; Van Bussel et al. 2006; Wallace and Gotlib 1990), the transition to grandparenthood has not attracted extensive research attention. It may be that becoming a grandparent seems like a trivial experience in comparison to the dramatic change of becoming a parent, which involves the recruitment of a wide range of resources and demands adaptation at all levels (Glade et al. 2005). Indeed, for a long time, the transition to grandparenthood was perceived solely as a happy event that required no coping or adaptation of any sort.

L. Findler and O. Taubman – Ben-Ari, *Grandparents of Children with Disabilities*, SpringerBriefs in Well-Being and Quality of Life Research,
DOI 10.1007/978-3-319-45517-4_2

The sparse scholarly interest in this life event might also stem from sociodemographic and sociocultural changes. Given the longer life expectancy in recent years, grandparents spend more time in this role, and take an active and meaningful part in their grandchildren's life, than in past years (Muller and Litwin 2011). Additionally, in recent decades, the family structure has undergone considerable change: more mothers are working full-time, divorce rates have risen, and there are more single-parent families by choice. These circumstances lead to a higher need for grandparents' help. Relying on grandparents' assistance has become increasingly common in the United States, England, and Australia, as has the phenomenon of grandparents raising their grandchildren as surrogate parents (Lumby 2010).

In addition, the study of development in older age in general is relatively new (Kallio and Pirttilä-Backman 2003). Although the contemporary approach holds that development occurs throughout the life course (Elder et al. 2003), not ceasing at the age of 18, the majority of developmental studies continue to relate exclusively to youngsters and young adults. Consequently, they ignore the fact that the extended lifespan and the new roles adopted in later stages of adult life in modern society mean that people often become grandparents at a time when they are still working and active in a variety of other domains. This situation makes it imperative to explore the competing roles and burdens in later adult life (Muller and Litwin 2011; Silverstein and Marenco 2001).

This chapter seeks to shed light on the transition to grandparenthood from a variety of perspectives. Throughout the chapter, we present the voices of the grandparents themselves, offering some of the thoughts and experiences they have shared with us in our studies. However, before focusing on specific characteristics of the transition to grandparenthood, we would like to consider certain aspects of life transitions in general.

2.1 Transitions Throughout the Lifespan

As noted above, research into adult development is relatively new (Elder et al. 2003; Kallio and Pirttilä-Backman 2003). Initial developmental theories related to infancy, early childhood, and adolescence, but paid little attention to later periods. Two of the most prominent theoreticians, whose influence on psychology is undeniable, are Sigmund Freud and Jean Piaget. Freud's psychoanalytic model consists of five psychosexual developmental stages (oral, anal, phallic, latency, and genital), the last of which occurs around the age of 13 (Freud 1905). Similarly, Piaget posited four stages of cognitive development, (sensorimotor, preoperational, concrete operational, and formal operational), with the last beginning around the age of 11 (Piaget 1952). More recently, along with the emerging understanding that individuals continue to develop in adulthood as well, developmental psychologists have added another stage, postformal thought, to characterize cognition at a later age (Kallio and Pirttilä-Backman 2003). Despite this addition, the underlying assumption of both theories is that individuals develop through a certain progression in their early years, and this development determines the rest of their lives, shaping their personalities, emotions, and behavior.

Erik Erikson, a follower of Freud, was the first eminent theoretician to relate to developmental stages throughout the lifespan, formulating a psychosocial model consisting of eight stages running from infancy to late adulthood. The three final stages relate to the mature periods (Erikson 1985).

According to Erikson (1985), in each stage, the individual has to cope with a "developmental crisis," and the manner in which this crisis is resolved influences coping with the next stage. In the middle adulthood, the central developmental challenge is the conflict between investment in oneself and responsibility and commitment to family and society. Those who resolve this conflict so that they experience caring and concern for others will be better able to cope with old age. Erikson contended that the fear of death is lower when a person has a sense of continuity and immortality through children. From this perspective, it is reasonable to assume that the way a person experiences the transition to grandparenthood and his or her readiness for the new role depends on the resolution of previous developmental crises and conflicts.

Along with the assumption that the way one copes with each of the developmental challenges is influenced by earlier stages and affects future ones, modern scholars claim a person's life may be viewed in terms of interactions between the various transitions they have gone through over the course of time (Perrig-Chiello and Perren 2005). Early transitions are considered particularly critical, impacting on life events that occur many years later. In other words, significant transitions that take place at an early age are definitive for later behavior (Elder 1998). Indeed, it has been found that normative life events and transitions predict several aspects of the well-being of middle-aged and older individuals at every point in time (Ryff and Heidrich 1997).

It goes without saying that transitions involve change. A person is in a transitional stage when there is a turning point in their life that requires adaptation and affects psychological development, such as leaving home, choosing a job or career, getting married, becoming a parent, or retiring (Cowan 1991; Lang et al. 2006). The changes also relate to the individual's roles in life, which are now redefined or discarded in favor of new ones (Perrig-Chiello and Perren 2005).

The literature describes two kinds of transitions: normative, which are generally positive; and non-normative, which tend to be negative and undesired, such as unemployment, chronic disease, or accidents (Cowan 1991). As non-normative transitions are unexpected by definition, there is no time to prepare for them, which means that they require a special type of coping and adaptation. We concentrate here, however, on normative life events like the transition to grandparenthood, which is considered a natural and anticipated stage in life.

Furthermore, in contrast to life transitions which take place at a certain age in childhood, adolescence, or young adulthood, such as starting school, entering high school, or joining the work force, the transition to grandparenthood occurs within a wider and more flexible age range. This highlights the importance of the socio-cultural element, in addition to the biological, in determining the age at which a life transition may take place (Perrig-Chiello and Perren 2005). Society sets norms for the appropriate timing for each transition, and by doing so gives meaning to events and their function in the lifespan. This "social time" relates to the length and sequence of roles, as well as to expectations and beliefs about each age and role in life. For example, a person may be said to marry "early" or "late" (Elder 1994). Similarly, the transition to grandparenthood may occur at an age that accords with or diverges from social expectations. Moreover, unlike most transitions, the age at which an individual becomes a grandparent is dictated by the plans of their children, and thus there is an uncontrollable element inherent in this event.

As human development is not the product of biology and environment alone, individuals are capable of making choices and impacting their own development (Elder et al. 2003; Haase et al. 2012), particularly in adulthood. Adults in modern western societies can choose the family structure they wish to belong to, perhaps deciding to have a child before or without marrying their partner, to create a family with a same-sex partner, or not to share a household with their partner. In addition, the timing of the transition to parenthood is more of a personal choice than it was in the past, due in part to medical technologies which enable conception and childbirth at a later age. However, the transition to grandparenthood, as mentioned above, is not at all a matter of personal choice, but is dictated by the deliberate life transition of another person, the son or daughter who decides to become a parent. This element is quite unique in adult life. Although usually viewed as a positive event, becoming a grandparent is essentially "forced" on the individual, regardless of whether or not they desire the role.

2.2 The Significance of the Timing of the Transition to Grandparenthood

The transition to grandparenthood is therefore an example of intergenerational dynamics, whereby a change in one generation affects another. As the lives of the family members are interconnected and mutually influential, the individual's development derives not only from the specific stage in their own life, but also from the developmental needs of other family members (Elder 1994). In the words of one grandfather:

> *I have a renewed understanding of what it means to be a young parent, and I enjoy the intergenerational continuity.*

The transition to grandparenthood is typically said to begin with the birth of the first grandchild. However, findings of a study on first grandmotherhood raise questions as to whether this is indeed the starting point, or whether the change actually begins earlier, during the mother's pregnancy. Examining a sample of mothers of daughters pregnant with their first grandchild, the study looked into the older woman's well-being and perception of the costs involved in the new role. The findings revealed no significant differences between grandmothers' reports in the third trimester of the pregnancy and two months after the birth of the grandchild (Ben Shlomo et al. 2010).

As noted above, the transition to grandparenthood takes place within a broad age range. However, the specific age at which it occurs appears to be significant. It has been found that adults who become grandparents at a younger or older age than the social norm report feeling older than peers who do so at what is considered the "appropriate" time in life. Thus, there appears to be a greater chance that the new role will be accepted more positively, with less ambivalence, difficulties, and conflict, when the transition occurs at the expected time. Furthermore, people who enjoy being grandparents report feeling younger, perceive aging as occurring at a later age, and hope to live longer than those who do not enjoy their role as grandparents (Kaufman and Elder 2003). These findings indicate that the transition to grandparenthood plays a meaningful role in the individual's age identity, that is, in whether people perceive themselves to be young, middle-aged or elderly. This effect is demonstrated in the following comments.

> *In a sense, the fact that I have a granddaughter enables me to relive previous experiences I had with my children, which makes me feel younger and older at the same time* (Grandfather).

> *Look, it makes me younger, yes, as many years have passed since I ran after my kids, barked like a dog, or pretended to eat them. And I haven't crawled on the floor or played with Lego, and it is fun to recall - not just to recall but to do everything again* (Grandfather).

Grandparents' age has also been related to the relationship they have with their grandchildren. Younger grandparents tend to live closer to their grandchildren and be more involved in assisting in their upbringing, while older grandparents tend to help more financially and identify more with the grandparental role (Silverstein and Marenco 2001). Age has been shown to be associated not only with grandparenting style, but also with life satisfaction, with younger grandparents reporting higher satisfaction (Ben Shlomo 2014). Thus, the age at which the transition to grandparenthood occurs appears to influence the grandparents' expectations and perceptions, which in turn affect the way the transition is experienced.

2.3 Experiencing the Transition to Grandparenthood

The transition to grandparenthood brings with it a shift in status, roles, and identities. It signals the start of a new stage in life, with the parenting role now supplemented by the role of grandparent (Kaufman and Elder 2003). Similar to other life transitions, it entails a great many changes, which may be experienced either positively or negatively.

The grandparent's relationship with the young grandchild has been found to be associated with a sense of achievement, meaning, and worth (Silverstein and Marenco 2001; Thiele and Whelan 2008). In addition, a positive perception of the role of grandparent has been shown to be related to higher self-esteem and a lower level of depressive symptoms (Reitzes and Mutran 2004), as well as to the wish to live longer, as noted above (Kaufman and Elder 2003). Grandmothers and grandfathers alike claim that none of their roles in adulthood has given them as much satisfaction as being a grandparent (Peterson 1999), and their enjoyment of the role is even greater than they expected before their grandchild was born (Somary and Stricker 1998). Grandmothers are happy to fulfill the role, and perceive it as a "second career" that affords them tremendous satisfaction and contentment (Gauthier 2002). The comments below illustrate this attitude.

> *The thought of my grandson makes me blissful and happy. I've felt much better since he was born* (Grandfather).

> *I'm more proud of my family, I dedicate more time to the family, I'm more at peace and happier with my life* (Grandfather).

In interviews with grandfathers, following the birth of their first grandchild, they described the difference between being a father and being a grandfather. As grandfathers, they are able to spend more time with their grandchildren than they had with their children, and are more involved than they were as fathers (Cunningham-Burley 2001; Sorensen and Cooper 2010). In addition, they have more patience with their grandchildren than they had with their children, attributing this not only to the greater amount of free time they have at their current stage in life, but also to the fact that they have less responsibility for the children, and have mellowed with age (Cunningham-Burley 2001). Moreover, grandchildren, and especially grandsons, enable grandfathers an emotional relationship and intimacy they seldom experienced with their own children (Sorensen and Cooper 2010). These differences are expressed in the following comments.

> *I have discovered that I have more energy and patience, I have become a softer person. I devote more time to my grandchildren at the expense of work, and often think about how I raised my own children* (Grandfather).

> *The relationship with my wife and children and with my granddaughter has become more meaningful and more intense. It's fun to play and spend time with a baby when I'm more settled and calmer than I was as a young father* (Grandfather).

Interviews conducted with Italian grandmothers produced similar findings, reflecting the significance of the role in their lives. They reported that the relationship with their grandchild afforded them emotional expression they had never experienced in any other relationship, enabled them to relive their role as mothers, and gave them an opportunity to correct the mistakes they had made with their own children. Like grandfathers, they also noted having more free time to enjoy the child than they had had as mothers (Gattai and Musatti 1999). Examples of grandmothers' comments appear below.

> *I had no idea it was possible for there to be such love. I didn't believe it. How can I love my granddaughters more than my own children? No, it's not that I love them more, it's that I feel more.*

> *There are four stages in life, and when a grandchild is born, you go one level up. You can see better from the tower.*

> *It activated systems I didn't have with my children. I mean, it's different, definitely different...With the grandchildren you're more mature, much more grown up in many ways, not just one. So your starting point is different, completely different. You're much more available, you're not angry any more. With your children you tend to be angry, that's how I felt, and here everything is possible. I mean, not that there's chaos, not at all, but your whole attitude comes from a completely different place, it's different.*

Numerous studies report the positive consequences of the transition to grandparenthood, some even claiming that becoming a grandparent has the most positive overall emotional valence of all transitions, followed by becoming a parent (Perrig-Chiello and Perren 2005). Nevertheless, positive affect may not be the only outcome. As with any transition, becoming a grandparent also entails the loss of previous identities and roles, as well as a variety of costs. In an Israeli study of grandmothers, the respondents reported both positive and negative thoughts and feelings. Higher active involvement with the grandchild was related to higher mental health among the grandmothers, but also to a higher perception of the costs involved in their role (Ben Shlomo et al. 2010). Given that the transition to grandparenthood generally takes place some time between the ages of fifty and sixty, a period considered young in modern society, the burdens on grandparents are considerable. Often they are still working, with some at the peak of their professional careers, they may have children living at home with them, they have social responsibilities and established leisure time activities, and now they are also expected to help care for their grandchildren and be involved in their nurturing. This burden may be very heavy, and result in complex personal and intergenerational tensions.

Negative emotions might also be aroused due to the fact that grandparenthood is symbolically associated with old age (Gauthier 2002), regardless of the chronological age of the individual or their level of vitality and activity. As Western society holds negative attitudes towards aging and views it as a threat (Perrig-Chiello and Perren 2005), acknowledging the process is painful, and involves awareness of unfulfilled hopes and expectations and limitations on future opportunities (Issroff 1994). These feelings may project on the way a person perceives their transition to grandparenthood.

Ambivalence toward the transition is apparent in psychoanalyst Issroff's (1994) description of her own experience:

> *I was struck by the extreme reactions of people when I told them I was about to become a grandmother. Either they said something like 'Oh, how wonderful' or 'You must feel so old'. Their responses confirmed the contradictory emotions that I felt. I felt narcissistically wounded by those who innocently asked me if this was my first and realized that I wanted to cling to the illusion that I didn't look like a grandmother. I was also aware of feeling out of control. Nobody asks you if you are ready to become a grandmother... As a relatively young grandmother I look forward to being able to watch and contribute to my grandson's growth and development, but his birth was a reminder that an era of my life is over. At the same time I was aware of many positive feelings - pride, pleasure, joy, and gratitude. Gradually I was able to acknowledge my ambivalence and think about the meaning of the feelings evoked by this important life event* (pp. 260–261).

Nevertheless, the professional literature tends to ignore the negative features of becoming a grandparent, focusing almost exclusively on the positive aspects. Moreover, studies generally relate to grandparents solely as providers of support, not addressing their own needs at this time in their life. In this sense, research reflects the attitude in society: whereas there are numerous workshops and guidebooks for expectant parents, virtually no such assistance is available for future grandparents, nor is it deemed necessary. As can be seen above, however, this is not the case. Much like becoming a parent, the transition to grandparenthood is a complex experience. A holistic, multidimensional examination of this transition is therefore needed not only to provide a fuller understanding of it, but also to enable interventions aimed at preparing people more effectively for their new role.

2.4 Factors Affecting the Experience of the Transition to Grandparenthood

In addition to age, another sociodemographic feature that has been found to affect the experience of grandparenthood is gender: men and women assimilate the role at a different pace. Grandfathers report that it takes them longer to provide help, become involved, and derive meaning from their new status in the family. In the early stages, they feel their role is not sufficiently well-defined, and may prefer to wait until the grandchild is a little older before playing an active part in his or her life (Cunningham-Burley 2001). One possible reason for this gender difference is the conventional role division, whereby women are more responsible for the care of infants. Indeed, studies show that with the birth of the first grandchild, women find it easier and more natural to step into the role of grandparent. Grandmothers were found to be more involved than grandfathers in caring for grandchildren (Silverstein and Marenco 2001), and to derive greater meaning and satisfaction from fulfilling this role. Whereas grandfathers feel capable of providing child-rearing advice to the parents, grandmothers report having to restrain themselves from giving too much advice in order to avoid the tension that might arise as a consequence (Somary and Stricker 1998).

A number of studies, however, have found no gender differences between grandparents on variables such as role satisfaction (Peterson 1999). This may be a reflection of changes in the grandfather's role in contemporary society. Recent studies indicate that grandfathers today are more involved and active in their grandchildren's lives, and may therefore perceive their role as more meaningful (Mann and Leeson 2010). Nonetheless, despite the increased involvement of grandfathers, significant differences in role perceptions persist. In a study conducted in Britain, for example, grandfathers themselves noted that grandmothers play a more important role in caring for the grandchildren, while their own activities with their grandchildren largely involve games, sports, and fun. In addition, grandfathers reported perceiving greater flexibility and freedom in respect to their role than grandmothers, having greater license to resist norms relating to commitment and involvement and to be critical of their children's functioning as parents and of their grandchildren (Mann and Leeson 2010). The disparities in the research findings may indicate that the shift in the perception of the grandfather's role is still a work in progress.

Another factor found to impact the grandparenting experience is whether the individuals are paternal or maternal grandparents. Lineage has been associated both with the nature of the interaction with the grandchild and with the sense of meaning derived from it (Somary and Stricker 1998). Maternal grandparents assist more in caring for their grandchildren (Wheelock and Jones 2002), and they also experience the transition to the new role as consisting of more challenges and threats alike, perhaps in view of the more central role they play (Ben Shlomo 2014).

Several studies suggest that the relationships between grandparents and their son- or daughter-in-law may be vulnerable, with the grandmother-daughter-in-law dynamic in particular being potentially conflictual (Rittenour and Soliz 2009), complex, and negative (Turner et al. 2006). Mothers tend to turn to their own mother for child-rearing advice, ignoring what their mother-in-law has to say (Marx et al. 2011). They are more likely to ask for help from their mother as well (Gauthier 2002). Nevertheless, the relationship with the father's parents can also be close and meaningful (Santos and Levitt 2007), with both sides providing support to each other (Rittenour and Soliz 2009). Moreover, a recent study examining life satisfaction following the transition to maternal and paternal grandparenthood found no differences between the two groups (Ben Shlomo 2014).

It should be noted that the majority of the literature focuses on maternal grandmothers due to their more central role and the strong connection with their daughter (Somary and Stricker 1998). As a rule, the mother-daughter relationship is highly significant, and often becomes even closer and more meaningful after the daughter gives birth (Marx et al. 2011). Mothers report that the support they receive from their own mother is extremely important to them (Scelza 2011), and such support has, in fact, been shown to be associated with higher well-being among new mothers (Taubman – Ben-Ari et al. 2009). This situation may lead naturally to a stronger relationship between the maternal grandmother and the grandchild.

Lineage has also been found to influence role expectations. Paternal grandfathers and grandmothers expect to see their grandchild less frequently than maternal grandparents (Somary and Stricker 1998).The latter finding is significant, as frequency of meetings with the grandchild has been shown to be related to grandparents' role satisfaction: the more frequent the meetings, the higher the satisfaction (Peterson 1999).

2.5 Grandparents' Well-Being During the Transition to Grandparenthood

As illustrated by the comments below, many grandparents describe positive feelings during the transition to their new role, including enjoyment, satisfaction, pride, happiness, and contentment.

> *... a sense of pride, great happiness, and awe* (Grandfather).
>
> *I became a grandmother just when I retired, earlier than expected, due to health problems. The combination of the two made it easier for me to go through this double transition. When I'm around my granddaughter, I feel totally healthy, young, and happy. During the week, I look forward to seeing her. I want to follow her development, to have time to enjoy watching her grow up* (Grandmother).
>
> *A feeling of satisfaction and enormous happiness, concern, feeling of closeness to a member of my family – a sense of liberation* (Grandfather).
>
> *New energy, a new joy in life, new spirit* (Grandfather).

Various studies have sought to identify factors that may contribute to mental health in the transition to grandparenthood (e.g., Ben Shlomo et al. 2010). Although life transitions center around change, research has shown that the best predictors of successful coping are the individual's characteristics prior to the transition (Cowan 1991). Clearly, the better the mental health of the individual, the more likely they are to assume a new role in life with less turmoil and to view it as a positive event. Recent studies conducted in Israel have identified several factors, including sociodemographic, personality, and environmental features, which were associated with the mental health of individuals who became grandparents in the previous two years.

In respect to sociodemographic characteristics, physical health was found to be particularly important, with better physical health associated with better mental health (Ben Shlomo et al. 2010; Ben Shlomo and Taubman – Ben-Ari 2012) and greater life satisfaction (Ben Shlomo 2014). This is not surprising, as older age brings with it more health problems, and even those who are currently healthy are aware that good health can not be taken for granted. Economic status was also found to be a relevant factor, so that the better grandparents' economic status, the better their mental health (Ben Shlomo 2014; Ben Shlomo and Taubman – Ben-Ari 2012).

In regard to personality traits, studies indicate the prime importance of self-esteem. Self-esteem is defined as an individual's global perception of self, whether positive or negative, and includes self-worth, pride, and self-acceptance (Rosenberg 1979). The Israeli studies found that higher self-esteem was related to higher mental health and a lower perception of the costs involved in the transition among first-time grandmothers (e.g. Ben Shlomo et al. 2010). It is likely that higher self-esteem provides an individual with a sense of security, thereby protecting them from the feelings of anxiety and upheaval that may be aroused by the new role.

Sense of mastery was also shown to be related to new grandparents' mental health, so that the higher the sense of mastery, the better the mental health (Ben Shlomo et al. 2010; Ben Shlomo and Taubman – Ben-Ari 2012). Finally, greater optimism was associated with grandparents' mental health, similar to the association between this personality trait and adaptation to other life transitions (Ben Shlomo and Taubman – Ben-Ari 2012).

In the case of environmental features, it is important to note that the empirical literature generally views grandparents as the providers of support, ignoring the fact that they too need a support system in order to maintain their mental health. Indeed, the studies found that a higher perception of receiving support was related to better mental health among new grandparents (Ben Shlomo and Taubman – Ben-Ari 2012). Furthermore, new grandparents who perceived better family ties reported higher life satisfaction (Ben Shlomo and Taubman – Ben-Ari 2016).

Like any life transition, becoming a grandparent is liable to generate costs. It involves taking on tasks that may be experienced as burdensome, as well as meeting the expectations of other family members and of the grandparents themselves. Coping with the new challenges may put a strain on available resources, create new problems, amplify existing limitations and sensitivities, and lead to tension and anxiety. At the same time, however, it may also enable the development of new coping capabilities and a higher level of adaptation (Cowan 1991; Cowan and Cowan 1995). This potential is defined by theoreticians as personal growth.

2.6 Personal Growth Following the Transition to Grandparenthood

> Since the birth of my grandson, I feel calmer and more relaxed, especially when I'm with him. My priorities have also changed; I devote more attention to my family at the expense of work, for example (Grandfather).

The term "personal growth" relates to positive psychological change that is experienced as a result of coping with challenging, and sometimes difficult, life events (Tedeschi and Calhoun 1996). The concept was originally introduced to describe the response to traumatic events that destabilize the individual's existing worldview and apprehension of their place in the world. In recent years, however, numerous studies have indicated that growth can also ensue from normative life events, such as the transitions to motherhood (e.g., Taubman – Ben-Ari et al. 2009, 2010), fatherhood (e.g., Spielman and Taubman – Ben-Ari 2009; Taubman – Ben-Ari et al. 2014; Taubman – Ben-Ari and Spielman 2014), and grandparenthood (e.g., Ben Shlomo et al. 2010; Taubman – Ben-Ari et al. 2012a, b). Events of this kind also call basic worldviews into question. When this leads to a process in which one's perceptions of life and self are reexamined and subsequently reconstructed in a more adaptive manner, enhancing the ability to cope efficiently with hardships and challenges, one can be said to evidence personal growth (Tedeschi and Calhoun 2004).

The process of growth entails both cognitive and emotional aspects (Zollner and Maercker 2006). It is reflected in three major domains: a change in self-perception, resulting in a sense of greater inner strength and a heightened ability to rely on oneself and cope with negative life events; a change in the perception of one's relationships with others, whereby relationships become more meaningful and one has a greater capacity to gain from them; and a change in life philosophy, in the form of a greater appreciation of life and a change in priorities (Tedeschi and Calhoun 1996). In other words, people who experience personal growth do not simply "overcome" an event, returning to the way they were prior to it, but rather develop in the wake of the event, becoming better adjusted, gaining more awareness of the meaning of life, and displaying healthier psychological functioning (Zollner and Maercker 2006).

It is important to bear in mind that although growth is a positive experience, it is not necessarily accompanied by improved well-being or a lower level of distress (Tedeschi and Calhoun 2004). No systematic associations have been found between growth on the one hand and characteristics of mental health on the other, including depressive symptoms, anxiety, anger, avoidance, self-esteem, meaning in life, and adaptation, among others (Zollner and Maercker 2006). This may be explained by the fact that personal growth does not reflect changes in well-being in the sense of affective state and hedonic enjoyment of life, but rather genuine development in terms of the understanding of one's role in life acquired through construction of a sense of meaning and commitment to the challenges encountered in the course of life (Joseph and Linley 2008).

In a recent series of studies conducted in Israel on personal growth following the transition to grandparenthood, new grandparents reported feelings and thoughts that indicate a process of growth, including changes in self-perception, interpersonal relationships, and priorities (Taubman – Ben-Ari 2012; Taubman – Ben-Ari and Ben Shlomo 2014). Changes in self-perception are reflected, for example, in comments like those below, which show that grandparents have discovered traits and abilities of which they were unaware prior to the birth of their grandchild.

> *There was a large hole that is filled up by this role. I'm happy and delighted to be around her. I'm like a lover! I miss her and I'm always looking forward to seeing her because it fills this big space in my life. I feel wanted, loved, and needed. My self-esteem is much higher now.* (Grandmother).

> *Back then, there wasn't this whole issue of expressing feelings like there is today. Today I have learnt from my children and I communicate with them much more, hugging and kissing them. The family is extremely important to me... I discovered my sensitivity and emotionality. I didn't know how much sensitivity there is in me; they've drawn it out of me. All this hugging, it's so moving. It's strengthened my understanding of how strong I am and how capable of achieving whatever I want* (Grandfather).

Grandparents also feel they have been given an opportunity to correct mistakes they made as parents, as evidenced in the following remarks.

> *The transition to grandmotherhood enabled me to come to terms with my parenthood and maybe gives me another chance to give, to influence, and to become a significant person in my grandchildren's lives.* (Grandmother).

> *I feel that my relationship with my granddaughter comes from a calmer and more mature place than the relationship I had with my children* (Grandmother).

In addition, grandparents' stories demonstrate improvement in personal and familial relationships following the transition to grandparenthood. They refer to the strengthening of their relationship with their children and their grandchildren, and the satisfaction and meaning these relationships afford them. Furthermore, they feel they have become part of "the community of grandparents", and some also note the cementing of their relationship with their spouse. The change in interpersonal relationships is apparent in the comments below.

> *My mood has improved, my relationship with my partner is better, I have more patience and tolerance for many things, a general feeling of serenity and forbearance* (Grandfather).

> *I think that being a grandmother caused my husband and me to be together in a new and special way, something very strong. Today we are sharing an experience which gives us a lot of joy, and it leads to a strong bond between us* (Grandmother).

> *Another dimension has been added to my life. I have something new in common with some of my friends, and I have another person to care for and think about. I feel unconditional love for my granddaughter* (Grandmother).

Finally, changed priorities, new goals in life, and a new outlook on life are all reflected in grandparents' comments. They talk about a new sense of pride derived from knowing they can help shape the young generation and serve as a role model to them. As can be seen below, they also note acknowledging their children as grown-ups with the change of their status to parents.

> *I'm more sensitive and open to the family and to others, proud of what I have achieved – my family and my granddaughter. I feel that I can, and must, be a model for her* (Grandfather).

> *I have less free time today, because much of my time is spent with my grandson. My attitude to my grandson is softer; I'm less concerned about teaching him how to behave. I have a stronger feeling of responsibility for the extended family, a stronger perception of my son as a person with his own family* (Grandfather).

Another interesting point raised by grandparents is the difference between the relationship they had with their children and the one they establish with their grandchildren.

> *The most pronounced change is the memory of raising my children that comes back to me. It's very refreshing to recall how it was. In addition, my perspective about children's upbringing has changed. Bringing up children means being on the inside, and with my granddaughter I get an interesting view from the outside. It makes me want to continue being involved in her life, and curious about what will happen with her in the future. It's different from raising children, when you concentrate very much on the present and you have no time to look into the distance. I'm very impressed and proud that my granddaughter is so close to me, and don't quite understand what I have done to earn this huge love of hers. I have so much fun with her, and so I do my best to make time for it on a regular basis* (Grandfather).

In addition to the studies that found personal growth among grandparents by means of self-reports acquired by questionnaires or interviews, two studies questioned another family member, either the spouse or offspring, regarding changes in the grandparent following the birth of the first grandchild (Taubman – Ben-Ari and Ben Shlomo 2014). Associations were found in these studies between grandparents' reports and the reports of significant others, indicating that personal growth is an experience that can be detected and acknowledged by people close to the individual.

The evidence of the potential to experience growth among grandparents raises the question of what factors might enable growth. Studies have examined several possibilities, including grandparents' sociodemographic characteristics, inner resources such as their personality traits, and external resources such as their marital relationship.

Similar to its role in the experience of becoming a grandparent, gender was also found to be associated with personal growth following the transition, with grandmothers reporting higher growth than grandfathers (Taubman – Ben-Ari et al. 2013, 2014). This may result from the difference in role perception and satisfaction between men and women, as described above. As the role of grandmother is perceived to be more central and significant, it may lead to a more profound developmental change, that is, to greater personal growth.

Age was also found to be related to personal growth, but only among grandmothers, with older grandmothers reporting higher growth (Taubman – Ben-Ari et al. 2012, 2013). This, too, may be linked to their greater involvement, which is likely to bring with it more difficulties and burdens than those of grandfathers. In addition, older age may increase concerns about health problems and physical limitations, as well as awareness of the time that has passed since the woman herself was a mother, thereby heightening her anxiety, which in turn may enhance the possibility of growth. In line with this explanation, one study found an association between lower health status and higher growth among grandmothers (Taubman – Ben-Ari et al. 2013).

Finally, an association was found between fewer years of education and higher growth among both grandparents (Taubman – Ben-Ari et al. 2013), similar to findings reported for mothers (Taubman – Ben-Ari et al. 2010). All these sociodemographic characteristics represent less favorable circumstances which may lead to greater tension and anxiety, and therefore may facilitate growth. As explained above, personal growth is a positive change that occurs as a consequence of coping with hardship. It may be assumed that the more difficult an individual's circumstances, the harder it will be for them to cope with the added burdens entailed in the transition to grandparenthood. As the challenge is greater, the sense of pride, accomplishment, and satisfaction derived from successfully managing it will also be greater. Such a process of positive change and learning on the new strengths and capabilities may stem from coping with the new role of grandparenthood.

As for internal resources, one of the personality traits that has been measured is grandparent's self-esteem. It was found that lower self-esteem among grandmothers was related to higher personal growth (Taubman – Ben-Ari et al. 2012a, b, 2014). This is similar in essence to the results obtained for the sociodemographic characteristics. Thus, like individuals who are older or less educated, those with lower self-esteem who successfully cope with the challenge of becoming grandparents might discover new qualities or abilities in themselves, leading to a sense of personal growth.

In respect to external resources, it was found that grandparent's personal growth was associated with that experienced by their spouse (Taubman – Ben-Ari et al. 2013). This suggests that the spousal relationship may enhance the possibility of a positive change by enabling the individual to share the meaningful experience of grandparenthood. Another factor found to be associated with growth among grandmothers is the frequency of meetings with the daughter who has recently become a mother (Taubman – Ben-Ari et al. 2012a, b). This measure might indicate either of a good mother-daughter relationship to begin with, or the opportunity to establish a better relationship between the two women than before the birth of the grandchild. In addition, higher meeting frequency most likely reflects greater involvement and commitment to the daughter, as well as a closer relationship with the grandchild. Similarly, among grandfathers, the frequency of meetings with the grandchild was positively associated with personal growth (Ben Shlomo and Taubman – Ben-Ari 2016). This may stem from significantly relationship which requires higher commitment and coping with the grandfather role.

External resources, in the form of the support system available to the individual, allow them to share feelings, receive emotional and instrumental support, and feel secure. This, in turn, enables them to develop a more adaptive perception of the new challenges they are facing (Cryder et al. 2006; Tedeschi and Calhoun 2004). Knowing that during challenging periods in life, which demand a reorganization and reconstruction of reality, there are significant others who will be at your side and share the difficulties with you is an essential and crucial part of the growth experienced in the transition to grandparenthood.

Taken together, the findings yielded by these studies indicate that lower personal resources and higher external resources facilitate the experience of growth among new grandparents. Moreover, they are in line with the results of investigations examining growth among women during the transition to motherhood (Taubman – Ben-Ari et al. 2009).

Most importantly, the studies demonstrate that a process of positive change occurs, at least among some individuals, in the wake of the transition to grandparenthood. Not surprisingly, however, if we compare the level of personal growth experienced by first-time parents with that of first-time grandparents, we find higher growth among new parents. The difference may stem from the fact that although the transition to grandparenthood is a significant life event, it is less dramatic than the transition to parenthood, and involves less momentous challenges (Taubman – Ben-Ari et al. 2012a, b, 2014). This does not diminish the importance of the transition to grandparenthood for the individual, but merely indicates a lower inherent potential for change than in the transition to parenthood.

Above all, the finding of growth among grandparents demonstrates the considerable significance of this role in life as a trigger for changes in perceptions of the self, interpersonal relationships, and indeed, life in general. It also indicates that this life transition, although positive in nature, also generates stress and necessitates coping. The positive change that may ensue as a result of the need to reexamine one's life, that is, personal growth, actually occurs because of the complex challenges posed by the new role.

To conclude, the transition to grandparenthood appears to be second in significance only to the transition to parenthood in adult life. In modern Western society, the role of grandparent has become even more central in the wake of sociodemographic and socioeconomic changes, as well as the acceptance of a multiplicity of family structures. Although current knowledge of the processes involved in the transition to grandparenthood is incomplete, both clinicians and researchers are displaying growing interest in the subject. It is hoped that further investigations will not only increase our theoretical understanding of how people cope with this life event, but will ultimately inform counselling and interventions, both on the individual and family levels, as well.

References

Ben Shlomo, S. (2014). What makes first time grandparents more satisfied with life? *Stress & Health, 30*, 23–30.

Ben Shlomo, S., & Taubman – Ben-Ari, O. (2012). New grandparents' mental health: The protective role of optimism, self-mastery, and social support. *Journal of Family Social Work, 15*, 274–281.

Ben Shlomo, S., & Taubman – Ben-Ari, O. (2016). What factors may assist social workers to promote life satisfaction and personal growth among first time grandfathers? *Child & Family Social Work*. doi:10.1111/cfs.12267

Ben Shlomo, S., Taubman – Ben-Ari, O., Findler, L., Sivan, E., & Dolizki, M. (2010). Becoming a grandmother: Maternal grandmothers' mental health, perceived costs, and personal growth. *Social Work Research, 34*, 45–57.

Cowan, P. A. (1991). Individual and family life transitions: A proposal for a new definition. In P. A. Cowan & E. M. Hetherington (Eds.), *Family transitions: Advances in family research series* (pp. 3–30). Hillsdale, NJ: Lawrence Erlbaum Associates.

Cowan, C. P., & Cowan, P. A. (1995). Interventions to ease the transition to parenthood: Why they are needed and what they can do. *Family Relations, 44*, 412–423.

Cowan, C. P., Cowan, P. A., Heming, G., Garrett, E., Coysh, W. S., Curtis-Boles, H., et al. (1985). Transition to parenthood: His, hers, and theirs. *Journal of Family Issues, 6*, 451–481.

Cryder, C., Kilmer, R., Tedeschi, R., & Calhoun, L. (2006). An exploratory study of posttraumatic growth in children following a natural disaster. *American Journal of Orthopsychiatry, 76*, 65–69.

Cunningham-Burley, S. (2001). The experience of grandparenthood. In A. J. Walker, M. Manoogian-O'Dell, L. A. McGraw, & D. L. G. White (Eds.), *Families in later life: Connection and transitions* (pp. 92–99). Thousand Oaks, CA: Pine Forge Press.

Elder, G. H. (1994). Time, human agency, and social change: Perspective on the life course. *Social Psychology Quarterly, 57*, 4–15.

Elder, G. H. (1998). The life course as developmental theory. *Child Development, 69*, 1–12.

Elder, G. H., Johnson, M. K., & Crosnoe, R. (2003). The emergence and development of life course theory. In J. T. Mortimer & M. J. Shanahan (Eds.), *Handbook of the life course* (pp. 3–19). New York, NY: Plenum Publishers.

Erikson, E. H. (1985). *The lifecycle completed: A review*. New York, NY: W.W. Norton & Co.

Freud, S. (1905). Three essays on the theory of sexuality. *SE, 7*, 125–245.

Gattai, F. B., & Musatti, T. (1999). Grandmothers' involvement in grandchildren's care: Attitudes, feelings, and emotions. Family relations: An interdisciplinary. *Journal of Applied Family Studies, 48*, 35–42.

Gauthier, A. (2002). The role of grandparents. *Current Sociology, 50*, 295–307.

Glade, A. C., Bean, R. A., & Vira, R. (2005). A prime time for marital/relational intervention: A review of the transition to parenthood literature with treatment recommendations. *The American Journal of Family Therapy, 33*, 319–336.

Haase, C. M., Heckhausen, J., & Wrosch, C. (2012). Developmental regulation across the life span: Toward a new synthesis. *Developmental Psychology, 49*, 964–972.

Issroff, R. (1994). Becoming a grandmother: The third position. *British Journal of Psychotherapy, 11*, 260–266.

Joseph, S., & Linley, P. A. (2008). Positive psychological perspectives on posttraumatic stress: An integrative psychosocial framework. In S. Joseph & P. A. Linley (Eds.), *Trauma, recovery, and growth* (pp. 3–20). Hoboken, NJ: Wiley.

Kallio, E., & Pirttilä-Backman, A. M. (2003). Developmental processes in adulthood–European research perspectives. *Journal of Adult Development, 10*, 135–138.

Kaufman, G., & Elder, G. H. (2003). Grandparenting and age identity. *Journal of Aging Studies, 17*, 269–282.

Keizer, R., & Schenk, N. (2012). Becoming a parent and relationship satisfaction: A longitudinal dyadic perspective. *Journal of Marriage and Family, 74*, 759–773.

Lang, F. R., Reschke, F. S., & Neyer, F. J. (2006). Social relationships, transitions, and personality development across the life span. In D. K. Mroczek & D. L. Todd (Eds.), *Handbook of personality development* (pp. 445–466). Mahwah, NJ: Lawrence Erlbaum Associates.

Lumby, J. (2010). Grandparents and grandchildren: A grand connection. *International Journal of Evidence-Based Healthcare, 8*, 28–31.

Mann, R., & Leeson, G. (2010). Grandfathers in contemporary families in Britain: Evidence from qualitative research. *Journal of Intergenerational Relationships, 8*, 234–248.

Marx, J., Miller, L. Q., & Huffmon, S. (2011). Excluding mothers-in-law: A research note on the preference for matrilineal advice. *Journal of Family Issues, 32*, 1205–1222.

Muller, Z., & Litwin, H. (2011). Grandparenting and psychological well-being: How important is grandparent role centrality? *European Journal of Ageing, 8*, 109–118.

Perrig-Chiello, P., & Perren, S. (2005). Biographical transitions from a midlife perspective. *Journal of Adult Development, 12*, 169–181.

Peterson, C. C. (1999). Grandfathers' and grandmothers' satisfaction with the grandparenting role: Seeking new answers to old questions. *International Journal of Aging and Human Development, 49*, 61–78.

Piaget, J. (1952). *The origins of intelligence in children*. New York, NY: International Universities Press.

Reitzes, D. C., & Mutran, E. J. (2004). Grandparent identity, intergenerational family identity, and well-being. *The Journals of Gerontology: Series B: Psychological Sciences and Social Sciences, 59B*, S213–S219.

Rittenour, C. E., & Soliz, J. (2009). Communicative and relational dimensions of shared family identity and relational intentions in mother-in-law/daughter-in-law relationships: Developing a conceptual model for mother in-law/daughter-in-law research. *Western Journal of Communication, 73*, 67–90.

Rosenberg, M. (1979). *Conceiving the self*. New York, NY: Basic Books.

Ryff, C. D., & Heidrich, S. M. (1997). Experience and well-being: Explorations on domains of life and how they matter. *International Journal of Behavioral Development, 20*, 193–206.

Santos, J. D., & Levitt, M. J. (2007). Intergenerational relations with in-laws in the context of the social convoy: Theoretical and practical implications. *Journal of Social Issues, 63*, 827–843.

Scelza, B. A. (2011). The place of proximity: Social support in mother-adult daughter relationships. *Human Nature, 22*, 108–127.

Silverstein, M., & Marenco, A. (2001). How Americans enact the grandparent role across the family life course. *Journal of Family Issues, 22*, 493–522.

Somary, K., & Stricker, G. (1998). Becoming a grandparent: A longitudinal study of expectations and early experiences as a function of sex and lineage. *The Gerontologist, 38*, 53–61.

Sorensen, P., & Cooper, N. J. (2010). Reshaping the family man: A grounded theory study of the meaning of grandfatherhood. *The Journal of Men's Studies, 18*, 117–136.

Spielman, V., & Taubman – Ben-Ari, O. (2009). Parental self-efficacy and stress-related growth in the transition to parenthood: A comparison between parents of pre- and full-term babies. *Health and Social Work, 34*, 201–212.

Taubman – Ben-Ari, O. (2012). Becoming and developing: Personal growth in the wake of parenthood and grandparenthood. In P. R. Shaver & M. Mikulincer (Eds.), *Meaning, mortality, and choice: The social psychology of existential concerns* (pp. 163–181). Washington, DC: American Psychological Association.

Taubman – Ben-Ari, O., & Ben Shlomo, S. (2014). Measuring the personal growth of new grandparents: A practical tool for social workers. Research on Social Work Practice, 1–8. doi:10.1177/1049731514564165

Taubman – Ben-Ari, O., Ben Shlomo, S., & Findler, L. (2012a). Personal growth and meaning in life in first-time mothers and grandmothers. *Journal of Happiness Studies, 13*, 801–820.

Taubman – Ben-Ari, O., Findler, L., & Ben Shlomo, S. (2012b). Personal growth and the transition to grandfatherhood. *The International Journal of Aging and Human Development, 74*, 265–285.

Taubman – Ben-Ari, O., & Spielman, V. (2014). Personal growth following the first child's birth: A comparison of parents of pre- and full-term babies. *Social Work Research, 38*, 91–106.

Taubman – Ben-Ari, O., Ben Shlomo, S., & Findler, L. (2014). First-time parents' and grandparents' perceptions of growth and their associations with self-esteem, cognitive appraisal, and social support: A dyadic approach. *Journal of Family Social Work, 17*, 229–250.

Taubman – Ben-Ari, O., Ben Shlomo, S., Sivan, E., & Dolizki, M. (2009). The transition to motherhood—A time for growth. *Journal of Social and Clinical Psychology, 28*, 943–970.

Taubman – Ben-Ari, O., Findler, L., & Ben Shlomo, S. (2013). When couples become grandparents: Factors associated with the growth of each spouse. *Social Work Research, 37*, 26–36.

Taubman – Ben-Ari, O., Findler, L., & Kuint, J. (2010). Personal growth in the wake of stress: The case of mothers of pre-term twins. *The Journal of Psychology, 144*, 185–204.

Tedeschi, R. G., & Calhoun, L. G. (1996). The posttraumatic growth inventory: Measuring the positive legacy of trauma. *Journal of Traumatic Stress, 9*, 455–471.

Tedeschi, R. G., & Calhoun, L. G. (2004). Posttraumatic growth: Conceptual foundations and empirical evidence. *Psychological Inquiry, 15*, 1–18.

Thiele, D. M., & Whelan, T. A. (2008). The relationship between grandparent satisfaction, meaning, and generativity. *The International Journal of Aging & Human Development, 66*, 21–48.

Turner, M. J., Young, C. R., & Black, K. I. (2006). Daughters-in-law and mothers-in-law seeking their place within the family: A qualitative study of differing viewpoints. *Family Relations, 55*, 588–600.

Van Bussel, J. C. H., Spitz, B., & Demyttenaere, D. (2006). Women's mental health before, during, and after pregnancy: A population-based controlled cohort study. *Birth: Issues in Perinatal Care, 33*, 297–302.

Wallace, P. M., & Gotlib, I. H. (1990). Marital adjustment during the transition to parenthood: Stability and predictors of change. *Journal of Marriage and the Family, 52*, 21–29.

Wheelock, J., & Jones, K. (2002). Grandparents are the next best thing: Informal child care for working parents in urban Britain. *Journal of Social Policy, 31*, 441–463.

Zollner, T., & Maercker, A. (2006). Posttraumatic growth in clinical psychology—A critical review and introduction of a two component model. *Clinical Psychology Review, 26*, 626–653.

Chapter 3
Being a Grandparent of a Child with a Disability

Liora Findler

Abstract When faced with the birth of a child with a disability, grandparents often experience a two-pronged crisis, feeling pain for their grandchild as well as for their own child. After the initial mourning process, most grandparents reconcile themselves to the situation and provide crucial emotional and instrumental support to the child and his/her parents. This chapter provides a grounded and nuanced picture of the experience of grandparents of children with disabilities as derived from the empirical and theoretical literature. It presents the voices of grandparents culled from interviews in which they reveal their personal feelings, insights, and experiences. In addition, it describes the complex intergenerational relationship and the delicate balance between involvement and interference in the life of the nuclear family. Finally, the chapter concludes with an innovative study that examined, for the first time, the possibility of personal growth among grandparents of children with disabilities.

Keywords Grandparenthood · Grandparents of children with a disability · Emotional support · Instrumental support · Personal growth · Positive psychology

Grandparenthood can be a very meaningful experience as it often offers a sense of immortality, a sense of continuity, and serves to compensate for past disappointments. Grandparents often perceive themselves as the torchbearers of the past and family legacy, history, rituals and customs. Grandchildren represent a link in the generational chain, and grandparents often see them as symbols of the future—those who will perpetuate their family line (Drew et al. 1998; Neugarten and Weinstein 1964). As such, the relationship between grandparents and grandchildren often carries with it an aura of exclusivity. Oftentimes, the grandparents' home is the place where three generations unite: grandparents, their children, and their grandchildren. A grandchild's progress and success can often be a source of pride and satisfaction for grandparents who see these accomplishments as confirmation of their success as parents, and as the 'dividend' they have earned from their investment in their children (Kivnick 1982; Neugarten and Weinstein 1964; Nybo et al. 1998).

L. Findler and O. Taubman – Ben-Ari, *Grandparents of Children with Disabilities*,
SpringerBriefs in Well-Being and Quality of Life Research,
DOI 10.1007/978-3-319-45517-4_3

The meaning associated with grandparenthood can create a set of expectations around the birth of a grandchild. These expectations may be challenged when a grandchild is born with a disability (Berns 1980; Seligman 1991). In general, the birth of a child with a disability often results in crises and challenges, which have lifelong implications on multiple aspects of family life (Bernier 1990; Wikler et al. 1981). Consequences include increased emotional, social, and financial pressures, alterations in family functioning, impairment of psychological well-being, and/or chronic distress (Florian and Findler 2001; Kazak and Christakis 1994; McCubbin and Patterson 1983; Wallander et al. 1990). These implications, and the need to cope with them, are not felt solely by the parents, but by other members of the nuclear and extended family as well, including the grandparents. As grandparents are often an essential part of a family's social support system, they are likely to experience the effects acutely. The birth of a grandchild with a disability often results in twofold distress for the grandparents who suffer the pain of the child and even more so, the pain of its parents, their own adult children (Anderson 2010a; Burns and Madian 1992; George 1988; Hall 2004; Seligman 1991; Woodbridge et al. 2009).

Despite the important position of grandparents in the family, and the recognition that raising children with disabilities impacts other family members, there is a paucity of research on the effects of a child with a disability on intergenerational relations (Seligman 1991; Vadasy 1987).

A review of the literature on families in crisis and family development reveals that for decades, grandparents have been marginal or negligible in discussions of families of a child with a disability. The sparse literature that exists regarding grandparents in such families focuses on the assistance and support they provide to their children and grandchildren, and not on the grandparents themselves (e.g. Findler 2000; Green 2001; Mirfin-Veitch et al. 1996, 1997; Mitchell 2008; Trute 2003). The personal experience of grandparents has yet to receive the research or clinical attention it deserves.

This chapter provides a review of the literature on grandparents of a child with a disability, and sheds light on the unique positions, experiences, and perspectives of these hidden family stakeholders. A comprehensive innovative study of grandparents' voices and experiences is included in this review (Findler 2009).

3.1 Contending the Diagnosis

It is documented in the literature that when a child is diagnosed with a disability parents often mourn the loss of their dream for a 'perfect' child, and are forced to cope with the consequent narcissistic injury (e.g., Hugger 2009; Riesz 2004; Whittingham et al. 2013). Grandparents often contend a similar experience; when a grandchild is diagnosed with a disability, grandparents are often caught unprepared, and are thus left feeling stunned and hurt. The diagnosis is often the starting pistol of an exhausting and emotional rollercoaster (Woodbridge et al. 2009). As described by a Grandfather of a child with a disability:

> *I've gone through a lot of hardship in my life even before this; it's not the first time I've been hurt. But when it comes to my granddaughter it's entirely different... it cuts you like an ax and there's no mental preparation for that... everything changes...*

When a child is diagnosed with a disability or illness, parents are often forced to be actively preoccupied with the many demands associated with the disability: physical care of the child, intensive meetings with doctors and other professionals, and adapting the home environment to the child's physical, cognitive, and emotional needs. Grandparents often undergo a mourning process similar to that of the parents, although from a more removed place (which may actually prolong the mourning period). Grandparents' distance from the day-to-day practical implications of dealing with the disability often leaves them only with a sense of loss. Furthermore, grandparents do not have access to the emotional and professional support and legitimacy offered to the parents, and often lack information regarding the nature of the disability and its short- and long-term ramifications (Anderson 2010b; Burns and Madian 1992; George 1988; Lee and Gardner 2010; Margetts et al. 2006). For example, in a study conducted by Katz and Kessel (2002), grandparents of a child with a disability expressed the feeling that the parents did not provide them with enough information about the child's diagnosis, or freedom to be involved in the child's daily routine. On the other hand, in another study, grandmothers reported that once they received specific information, they were able to better meet the needs of their grandchildren with disabilities (Gallagher et al. 2010).

A US study that examined the reaction of 32 grandparents to their grandchild's diagnosis of disability (Scherman et al. 1995) illustrated the total unpreparedness grandparents experienced and the way in which it made facing and accepting the reality more difficult. Specifically, although informed of the presence of the disability immediately after the birth, these grandparents were not given detailed information about the child's condition. Participants reported experiencing a sense of shock, loss, anger, denial, disgust, and uncertainty which were exacerbated by a lack of information and support.

As noted earlier, the pain the grandparents contend is two—or even three-fold: pain for themselves, pain for their children, and pain for their grandchild (Moules et al. 2012). The birth of such a child not only changes grandparents' daily routine and expectations, it may also shatter their fantasy of the future of their family. The pain grandparents feel for themselves is often related to narcissistic injury, disappointment, and even shame (Vadasy 1987).

A study by Findler (2009) examining the experience of grandparents of children with intellectual disabilities revealed that the initial diagnosis of disability aroused extremely strong and painful emotions which remained carved in their memories; at the time of the interviews which was years after the diagnosis, participants described the diagnosis and the feelings it aroused in vivid detail. Some participants acknowledged that their initial reaction was hope to spare their own adult children the difficulty of raising a child with a disability. To quote one grandmother:

> *From my point of view, it was a catastrophe that I couldn't simply accept... As I saw it, she [the mother] had lost her life. If he lived, she wouldn't live, or she'd have a very bad life.*

In some cases, the diagnosis of disability is given at birth or soon after. In other cases, the diagnostic process may be lengthy, prolonging the ability to cope with it. Even in circumstances in which the diagnostic processes was lengthy, several grandparents revealed uncertainty and a lack of understanding; they stated that they were aware that a problem had been discovered but were unable to provide details about the condition and its implications (Findler 2009).

On the other hand, some grandparents credited themselves for being active in, and even initiating, the diagnostic process. According to Anderson's report (2010a) many grandparents played a vital role in early recognition of their grandchild's ASD. Not only did nearly half the grandparents say they had provided support to a parent who was raising concerns, but also 30 % reported they were the first to notice a problem with their grandchild's development.

However, these grandparents, the ones who identified the presence of an issue before the parents realized, faced the additional dilemma of whether or not to broach the subject with their child, their grandchild's parent. Because of the sensitivity of the subject, and concern about the pain they would likely cause, grandparents expressed anxiety about the angry reaction that would be invoked by raising the issue. For example, one grandmother of a child with a disability discussed how she noticed impairments in her grandchild's development:

> *I knew right away that there was a problem...from experience. She didn't look at me, didn't make eye contact. She had the symptoms of autism...Right away I knew there would be a problem, I was sure of it. When I said so...she [the mother] got angry. She said, 'She is still very little, what do you want? You can't tell'. But I knew. I wasn't surprised by anything. They were all blind.*

Studies show that the majority of grandparents of a child with a disability are actively involved in the diagnostic process from the beginning (Anderson 2010b; Gallagher et al. 2010). However, the extent and nature of involvement vary; although some grandparents find it difficult to be supportive for their children as they are dealing with their own profound sorrow (Seligman 1991), most feel that at this difficult junction it is their duty to repress their own pain and feelings of distress and anxiety, in order to provide support for their children (Miller et al. 2012). Furthermore, grandparents were often involved in decisions for their grandchildren. In Anderson's report (2010b), more than 70 % said they had played some part in treatment decisions made for their grandchild, with 22 % saying they were very involved, or had even taken the lead on decisions regarding treatments.

3.2 Emotional Processing

Accompanying their children through the process of the diagnosis often arouses existential questions and uncertainties regarding injustice and fate among grandparents. Grandparents try to make meaning of the experience and to understand 'why' this had happened to them and to their family (Woodbridge et al. 2011). Moreover, grandparents' pain is often accompanied by fear and anxiety that their children will be too busy addressing the needs of the child and thus, will be unable to care for them in their old age (Findler 2009). These feelings are not socially legitimate and thus are not easily expressed.

In addition to the pain they feel for themselves, grandparents suffer emotionally for their children as well, as it can be particularly difficult to witness their children coping with such a challenging situation. In the words of a grandmother talking about her daughter and grandchild:

> *I was fighting for her life and she was fighting for his life. That's how it was. I was just fighting for her life. I said to myself that she didn't know what was waiting for her, that her married life, her romance, her joy in life, was over.*

The third pain grandparents experience is the emotional pain they feel for their grandchild. It is difficult for them to witness the pain their grandchild experiences, and imagine the pain the child will contend in the future. Grandparents are often concerned about the possibility that their grandchild with a disability, a child who is socially vulnerable, will be abused or injured (Findler 2009). The comparison with other children of a similar age is painful for grandparents at each stage in the child's development; each milestone in the child's life provides further evidence of the lost potential. In many cases, grandparents are distressed less by the actual disability and difficulties the child will face and more by what he or she will miss out and never get to know or achieve (Woodbridge et al. 2011). Additionally, while in typical circumstances, grandparents often anticipate a time when their grandchildren will be grown and independent, imagining the support and family continuity such a transition would provide, grandparents of a child with a disability don't have that luxury, and often fear for the child's fate once the child's parents grow old (Scherman et al. 1995).

3.3 Between Denial and Acceptance—Reactions to Child's Disability

In her study, Findler (2009) found a large extent of heterogeneity in the manner in which grandparents described their grandchild's disability. Some grandparents related primarily to the official diagnosis and its symptoms, others refrained from using the formal diagnosis, and instead depicted the specific problems (i.e.

difficulties in school or motor impairments). For example, a grandfather of a child with a disability stated:

He doesn't talk, and he doesn't hear very well either. He can't move one leg. He's fed through a tube. He's got a lot of problems.

Some grandparents are able to see beyond the disability and choose instead to focus on positive aspects of their grandchild without letting the disability overwrite their view of the child. These grandparents note developmental improvements or stress the uniqueness of the child despite the disability. In some cases, grandparents minimize the severity of the disability by emphasizing the love they have for the child and the special relationship they have with him or her. These grandparents often voice optimism concerning the future (Katz and Kessel 2002). However, this minimization, optimism, and positive outlook often mask denial; grandparents often attempt to normalize or minimize the child's difference instead of facing and/or embracing his/her disability. As a grandmother of a child with a disability described her grandson:

He's fine. It's just that other kids have a bad influence on him. He doesn't look odd or different, Heaven forbid.

This denial can be so great that these grandparents turn a blind eye to reality to the extent that they create fantasies about imaginary medications, paint an unrealistic picture of the disability, and/or adopt exaggerated optimism (Seligman 1991; Seligman et al. 1997).

Grandparents' difficulty in accepting a grandchild's disability and dealing with the consequent pain and disappointment may cause them to perceive the situation in an unrealistic light, seek explanations or justifications, or to deny the disability entirely. However, over time, most grandparents come to terms with the diagnosis and learn to cope in their own ways. Initial feelings of sadness, helplessness and anxiety give way to more positive feelings of acceptance, hopefulness and involvement (Schilmoeller and Baranowski 1998). According Anderson (2010a), grandparents occasionally felt they had, at some point, been in denial about their grandchild's ASD. Some of them on the other hand, felt their adult child, the grandchild's parent, had been in denial at some point, and even more indicated that their child's spouse had been in that state. Interestingly, grandparents were more likely to view sons or sons-in-law as having been in denial than daughters or daughters-in-law. Similarly, some of them reported their grandchild's other grandparents had had trouble accepting the child's diagnosis.

3.4 Adapting to the Unique Circumstances

Once a concrete diagnosis of a disability has been made, grandparents are confronted with the challenge of coping with the new reality and its implications on their families and their own lives. Schilmoeller and Baranowski (1998) studied grandparents of a child with cerebral palsy at the time of diagnosis and at a subsequent interval. They found that the negative emotions that grandparents experienced when they learned of the disability (i.e. anger, confusion, helplessness, and betrayal) were moderated over time. Specifically, further down the road (after the diagnosis), the negative emotions were replaced by more positive ones such as a sense of calm, hope, strength, vitality, and acceptance; the more the grandparents adapted to the new reality, the stronger these feelings grew. Similarly, a study by Findler (2009) found that grandparents of a child with a disability reported positive emotions and unconditional love for the grandchild:

> *My granddaughter... if they told me now to do the craziest thing on earth to give her comfort, joy, or pleasure, I'd do it. I'm not talking about her health, which I'd give parts of my own body for. It's unconditional love. There are no conditions to this love.*

Nonetheless, these positive feelings were often mixed with pain, concern, and sorrow. Gradual acceptance of the new reality of disability is a journey, one that begins with existential quandaries and continues with the reexamination and reframing of expectations of grandparenthood. This journey involves searching for and finding a meaningful answer to the question of "why us?" As grandparents reflect on the expectation of "ideal grandparenthood" and compare it with their own experience, they derive new insights and modify their expectations and definitions. Through this process they cast aside previous fantasies about the activities and interactions they expected to enjoy with their grandchild, replacing them with revised plans and expectations (Katz and Kessel 2002; Woodbridge et al. 2011).

3.5 Grandparenting a Child with a Disability: Navigating Styles, Roles and Meaning

The role of a grandparent of a child with a disability may take on a variety of forms and include the provision of instrumental, financial, and/or emotional assistance (Hillman 2007; Katz and Kessel 2002; Schilmoeller and Baranowski 1998). Woodbridge et al.'s study (2011) on 22 Australian grandparents of a child with a disability examined the classic typology of Neugarten and Weinsten (1964). Their findings indicate that participants adopted three out of the five grandparenting styles: "surrogate parent", "fun-seeking", and "reservoir of family wisdom". Most of these grandparents did not adopt the "formal" or "distant" grandparenting styles. Those who adapted a 'surrogate parenting' style felt that they were called upon to enhance the welfare and functioning of the nuclear family. They accompanied the parents to medical appointments and treatments, looked after their grandchildren for several hours or even days, and performed numerous other instrumental tasks. The role of 'reservoir of family wisdom' was performed by contributing to the grandchildren's knowledge and by teaching them and instilling cultural and traditional values (Woodbridge et al. 2011, p. 360). According to Woodbridge et al. (2011)

grandparents often saw their role as a conduit to other members of the family, both past and present, fulfilling an educational "kinkeeping" activity, role and style. Grandparents described the importance of maintaining wider family bonds, recalling how they would take their grandchildren to visit family, to the country and to go camping. Unfortunately, maintaining these family bonds was sometimes challenging, as wider family members struggled to cope with and accept the reality of disability.

The primary contribution of grandparents of a child with a disability is the instrumental and emotional support they provide (Hillman 2007). Although these types of support are features of 'grandparenting in general,' in the case of a child with a disability, they become more crucial and take on special meaning (Findler 2009). Whereas some of the activities these grandparents perform relate specifically to the child with a disability, others are more general and are meant to ease the burden on the parents to enable them the freedom to spend time with their spouse and other children or advance their careers (Scherman et al. 1995).

Instrumental support includes babysitting, chauffeuring, trips and outings, imparting knowledge, and assisting with homework (Gardner et al. 1994; Schilmoeller and Baranowski 1998). The importance of grandparents' instrumental support lies in providing a support system for concrete needs including medical care that requires an understanding of the complexity of the disability and the demands and treatment it entails. Indeed, after the shock of the initial diagnosis, some grandparents learn and display an impressive command of medical terminology, the physical implications of the disability, and the most effective treatment and intervention strategies for the child (Gardner et al. 1994). Another form of instrumental support that grandparents frequently provide is financial assistance intended to ameliorate the extended costs of the family (Anderson 2010b).

Emotional support is provided to the grandchild and his/her parents through listening, empathy verbal and physical expressions of unconditional love (hugs and kisses), praise for the grandchild, and playing with the child. Grandparents often express empathy and support for their child's feelings of sadness, frustration, or disappointment (Findler 2009). The emotional support they provide is significant as it is geared towards providing their adult child with someone to talk to, a sense of shared destiny, and the security to openly and honestly express their pain, frustrations, and disappointments without fear of being judged.

In many cases, grandparents of a child with a disability perceive their role as one that is a critical source of support and requires total commitment to the needs of their children and grandchildren. These grandparents often display a great deal of commitment to helping their adult child and their grandchild, regardless of age and physical limitations (Gardner et al. 1994; Schilmoeller and Baranowski 1998). They often feel that when their children are dealing with such difficult and demanding circumstances it is inappropriate for them to be concerned with their own needs (Findler 2009).

3.6 Personal Costs and Prices

The dedication and commitment of grandparents towards their children and grandchildren often comes at a price. The cost of supporting their family includes setting aside their own dreams, putting off plans to travel or indulge in hobbies, and working fewer hours in order to be closer and provide more help to their children (Woodbridge et al. 2011).

Research indicates that grandparents may also pay a social price. Specifically, Findler (2014) found that perceived social support from friends was lower among grandparents of a child with an intellectual disability in comparison with grandparents of children without a disability. This is consistent with findings about mothers of a child with a disability who report a smaller network of friends and acquaintances in comparison with mothers of children with typical development (Findler 2000). It appears that grandparents who devote themselves to their families find it hard to cultivate social relationships. Grandparents of a child with a disability can feel uncomfortable in the company of their peers, especially when the conversation turns to the development and achievements of their typically developing children and grandchildren. Not surprisingly, grandparents often prefer to avoid such situations. Additionally, unlike close family relationships which generally endure unusual events or circumstances, friendships that are not actively nurtured by both sides tend to fade (Findler 2009).

Grandparents are key figures in families of a child with a disability, and they often take upon themselves the unique role of preserving the family's quality of life and promoting its happiness (Miller et al. 2012). However, grandparents' advanced age may pose as a challenge as it often impedes their current functioning and serves as a constant reminder of the time when they will no longer be able to provide the emotional and instrumental support their family requires. In addition, grandparents are often torn between their own needs and those of the other members of the family. Striking a balance can be extremely difficult. As a result of this tension, many grandparents of a child with a disability choose to reject career opportunities and discard plans for retirement, instead preferring to be close to their children and offer them the help they need. It is important to note that grandparents do not always feel that their children are grateful for the significant effort they make (Miller et al. 2012).

The time and energy grandparents invest in the child with a disability may cause their other children and grandchildren to feel neglected. Dividing their resources fairly among all members of the family is proven to be difficult, and grandparents are liable to find themselves at the heart of a conflict saturated with envy and possessiveness (Miller et al. 2012).

Findings of Woodbridge et al. (2011) indicate that grandparents of a child with a disability often regard themselves as mediators within the extended family. As the presence of the child with a disability may adversely affect relations with members of the nuclear and extended family, grandparents often feel it is their duty to arbitrate and prevent the conflicts that may arise. In some cases, the first signs of conflict appear before the birth of the child and become more intense after the birth; in other cases conflict arises in the wake of the new reality. Heightened sensitivity to verbal comments or minor acts often leads to conflict, particularly at family events. Grandparents often feel caught between conflicting expectations—wishing to protect the child with the disability from unseemly reactions of aunts, uncles, or cousins, while at the same time maintaining their own close relations with them. Findler (2009) found that oftentimes at family gatherings grandparents are hurt when witnessing the isolation and ostracism facing their grandchild with a disability. They often feel that it is their responsibility to intervene to ensure the child gets sufficient attention from siblings and cousins. Similarly, Findler (2009) found that grandparents often feel obligated to develop exceptional sensitivity and balance to ensure that they are able to attend to the special needs of the child with a disability without neglecting their other grandchildren.

3.7 A Delicate Balance: Involvement versus Interference

The desire to provide support and be involved in the life of their grandchild often conflicts with grandparents' fear of interfering. The strong social and cultural mandate regarding the autonomy and independence of adult children (Johnson 1998), alongside the ill-defined status and ambiguous expectations of the grandparenting role in our society (Fischer and Silverman 1982), places grandparents in an internal conflict regarding their level of involvement. This delicate dilemma becomes particularly sensitive in the case of families of children with disabilities (Sullivan et al. 2012). Grandparents often find themselves walking a fine line in respect to their place within the lives of their children and grandchildren. They endeavor to support without being a burden, guide without being intrusive, and provide love and warmth without being cumbersome (Burns and Madian 1992). Even when they are actively involved in their grandchildren's care, grandparents are often hesitant to express their thoughts and feelings, and are even more reluctant to voice criticism of their children's parenting (Katz and Kessel 2002).

Recognizing the difference between the roles of grandparent and parent, grandparents typically walk on eggshells and think twice before intervening in the life of their child's family. Even if they feel that their children are neglecting their grandchildren, grandparents believe that they are not responsible for the child's upbringing and their role is to take a step back. Grandparents are usually sensitive to the "rules of the game" dictated by the parents, and do their best to abide by them. Should there be an argument between the parents and the children, or between the parents themselves, grandparents generally choose to keep their distance and not take sides (Findler 2009). It is important to note that while these issues are often found amongst all grandparents, with grandparents of a child with a disability, these issues may take on greater significance, sensitivity, and weight.

Findler (2009) points out that grandparents' restricted involvement is derived from their own recognition that they do not occupy center stage in the child's life.

This belief is reinforced by the messages they receive from their children concerning the limits of their role. In efforts to maintain good relations with their children and be considered as cherished members of the family, many grandparents maintain the boundaries set out for them (Findler 2009).

While some grandparents are aware of the limits of their authority and try to refrain from overstepping boundaries, others believe that the support they provide grants them certain rights and power. Specifically, they feel that their financial and instrumental assistance entitles them to express opinions and make suggestions regarding the upbringing of the grandchild with a disability (Findler 2009).

3.8 Negotiating Differences of Opinion

Grandparents' often hold different opinion than those of their children. There are a few central issues most likely to arouse grandparents' criticism amongst them, the way in which their children speak to their grandchildren, inappropriate diet, and lack of clear boundaries set for their grandchildren's behavior. In families of a child with a disability, the subject of the grandchild's special needs tends to cause the most conflict; grandparents often feel that the parents of the child with a disability respond inadequately to the child's needs, are negligent about treatment and/or diagnosis, and are lax in finding and/or trying to search for solutions to the child's issues (Findler 2009). At a later stage, post diagnosis, grandparents may have reservations about the educational institution in which the grandchild with a disability is placed, often believing it does not suit the child's level and/or needs. A few grandparents report feeling that the grandchild is not shown enough love by their parents (Findler 2009). The conflict grandparents face between wishing to be involved in their child and grandchild's lives and the fear of being blamed for interference may intensify as the child develops.

Grandparents cope with these differences in many ways including estrangement, constant criticism, completely backing down, and/or enduring any offense or acrimony in order to avoid damaging the relationship. For the most part, grandparents consider their words carefully and make efforts to choose their battles by setting priorities regarding issues that warrant a comment and issues that do not; attempts are made to choose suitable times to express opinions they do decide to vocalize. Some grandparents, particularly grandmothers, employ open dialogue as a problem-solving and conflict resolution strategy in order to build intergenerational relationships based on open communication, trust, and honesty (Findler 2009).

As discussed above, the moment when grandparents suspect that their grandchild is not developing typically, they are faced with a dilemma: on the one hand, grandparents know how important it is to make parents aware of a possible issue and encourage them to seek help as early as possible. On the other hand, they are often afraid to voice their concerns out of fear that they will cause their children pain and thus, be a target of their anger. Some grandparents feel that they do not have a close enough relationship with their child and thus, they do not have the openness to discuss concerns or interfere in their children's lives (Findler 2009). As a grandmother of a child with a disability expressed:

> *I don't know how they didn't see it...I saw immediately because of my experience as a mother that she didn't have the skills of a 13-month-old. None of them. Nothing. I saw it clearly, and all the time I felt they weren't doing enough to fix the problem. To this day they don't do enough.*

However, grandparents felt that voicing concern, criticism, or offering suggestions regarding the grandchild requires particular sensitivity. Specifically, although grandparents may recognize the importance of informing parents about medical assistance and/or treatment options, they are aware of the difficulty their children face and do not wish to add to their distress by making them feel incompetent or guilty.

The complexity of these circumstances is evident in participants' comments as a grandmother of a child with a disability stated:

> *I think that if they left the child with me more, she'd make more progress. There's no doubt in my mind. I'm not being judgmental. She is their first child, and there's the matter of possessiveness and exclusivity, and on top of that she is a child with problems. Looking at it from the side, I think that if they let her go a little more, she'd be less dependent on them and she'd develop more...I'm not going to bulldoze them. I know the puzzle, and I work within it. It was harder at the beginning. I worked on myself...just take a minute, be smart, you've only got one son, one granddaughter, one daughter-in-law. Work with them.*

There are times when grandparents feel a sense of urgency and take the initiative to seek solutions needed to support grandchild's development. Others attempt to relay the message to their children in an open and reasonable manner, and only if they come up against a brick wall do they feel they have to use force to get their point across. Other grandparents are more sensitive to the complexity of the situation, and thus display acute understanding of the parents' difficulties, recognizing that their criticism would be unconstructive, unfounded, and insensitive (Findler 2009). Despite these differences, many grandparents are involved and try easing the reality for their children and grandchildren by helping as much as possible. However, this help varies from family to family and from grandparent to grandparent.

3.9 Grandparents' Involvement and Support: Contributing Factors

There is a variety of factors contributing to the degree to which grandparents are involved in their children's families. These include interpersonal and familial relations (i.e. the relationship between the grandparents and their children, affectional solidarity); personal traits (i.e. gender and health), and structural factors (i.e. geographical distance).

3.9.1 Interpersonal and Familial Relations

The nature and history of the relationship between the grandparents and their children appear to have the most significant impact on the quality and character of the support grandparents offer their children. This is particularly true in unique circumstances, such as when a child is diagnosed with a disability. According to Mirfin-Veitch et al. (1996, 1997), the quality and components of the intergenerational connection in families of children with disabilities do not stem from the presence or severity of the grandchild's disability, but rather from the family relations prior to the birth. The authors contend that a history of family intimacy and open communication serve as the foundation for empathy and emotional and instrumental support after the birth of a child with a disability. In contrast, a history of emotional distance and relationships characterized by coldness and closed communication leads to estrangement and a lack of support.

Similarly, Schilmoeller and Baranowski (1998) examined predictors of grandparents support and involvement among seventy grandparents of children with cerebral palsy. The authors found that of all the dimensions of intergenerational solidarity delineated by Bengtson and Mangen (1988) and Bengtson and Roberts (1991) affectional solidarity (i.e. emotional exchanges between adult members of the family, the quality of their relationships, displays of love, affection) predicted the level of support grandparents of children with disabilities offered their offspring. (Schilmoeller and Baranowski 1998). Naturally, in families of children with disabilities, affectional solidarity took on unique significance as the parents might contend isolation and loneliness. However, in some cases, while grandparents felt capable of providing instrumental support, they found it difficult to offer emotional support for fear of interfering in sensitive issues and hurting their children (Schilmoeller and Baranowski 1998).

3.9.2 Gender Differences

Gender differences have been found in the type and level of grandparents' participation in the lives of their children and grandchildren, as well as the perception of the nature and quality of the intergenerational relationship. Gender can be related to grandparenthood through one of three routes: grandparent's gender, grandchildren's gender or maternal/paternal grandparent status. Grandmothers are often more involved in childcare, and as such, have more of a tendency to experience the family more intensely. Indeed, many of the grandmothers in Findler's (2009) study, identified their role as 'grandmother' as their mission in life, viewing themselves as a key figure in their children's' families.

In contrast, there are fewer social expectations of men to take on an active role in family life, either instrumentally or emotionally (Bates 2009). However, grandfathers who did not spend much time raising their own children because they had been busy building a career and financially supporting their family, often take great pleasure in doing with their grandchildren what they missed out on with their own offspring (Findler 2009). In other words, grandfatherhood can offer men the opportunity to compensate for their absence from family life when their children were young. According to Thomas (1986) in later years although women often continue their 'mothering' roles, the gender division of roles which is so prevalent when raising children becomes blurred and men often change, become gentler, and share more in family tasks.

The central role that women play in family life may also explain the special place often held by a daughter's family in contrast with that of their sons. It is not surprising that grandparents' preference for their daughter's family over their sons runs like a thread through empirical studies and clinical reports (e.g., Rossi and Rossi 1990). Grandparents often describe their relationship with their daughter and her children as stronger and a greater source of reward than their relationship with their son's family. Consequently, they tend to visit their daughter more often, feel more comfortable with her, and are not concerned that they may not be welcome or are interfering, as is often the case with their daughter-in-law (Seligman 1991).

The middle generation is commonly held responsible for the tri-generation relationship, with the mother being most active in the ties with the extended family (Katz and Kessel 2002). The relationship between a mother and her daughter-in-law is likely to be delicate and sensitive, as it marks an intimate encounter between two families that may represent different values, norms, and behaviors. By nature, it can be easier for the daughter in law to turn first to her own family of origin, particularly her mother for emotional and practical support. (Bowen 1978; Seligman et al. 1997). In general, the relationship between a woman and her spouse's family might be sensitive and vulnerable; under unique circumstances such as raising a child with a disability, the sensitivity of these relationships might be even greater.

According to Katz and Kessel (2002), grandparents' involvement in their grandchildren's lives was mostly determined by the parents desires, as any information regarding their grandchild's condition and its implications was entirely in the parents' hands. The parents of the fathers often reported feeling particularly constrained and dependent on the willingness of their daughter-in-law to share this information with them. In Findler's (2009) study as well, participants noted the different experiences they had in the relationships they had with their daughter's family in comparison with the relationship they had with their sons.

3.9.3 Health

Grandparents in poor health or advanced age often feel that the physical effort required to provide the necessary instrumental support (i.e. picking up their grandchildren, playing with them, feeding, bathing, or putting them to bed) is too difficult for them (Burns and Madian 1992). The care needs of a grandchild with a disability may be even more demanding and require greater effort. Grandparents report that they are often unable to do everything they would like to with the child because of limited physical abilities, age, and/or health (Shaw 2005).

3.9.4 Geographical Distance

Geographical distance greatly affects grandparents abilities to support their children. This challenge is felt particularly in the United States, where grandparents often reside in a different state from their adult children (e.g. Gardner et al. 1994; Nybo et al. 1998). Geographic distance often hinders grandparents' daily involvement in their grandchild's life, particularly regarding information sharing. Gardner et al. (1994) found that the frequency of meetings between grandparents and their children and grandchildren declines when they live more than a 30 or 45 min drive apart. In such cases, the grandparents are less open to learning how to care for their grandchildren, and often find it hard to make themselves available for routine tasks on short notice, which is often a great need. According Anderson (2010b), some grandparents who lived far away and were unable to play an active role felt guilty as well as sad that they did not have the day-to-day chance to learn to interact well with their grandchild with the disability.

A qualitative study of grandparents of a child with a hearing impairment (Nybo et al. 1998) found that although geographic distance was not found to impact grandparents relationship with their adult child as it was possible to obtain information and provide emotional support over the telephone, the distance led to communication problems with the grandchild who was unable to communicate by phone. The authors claim that extreme geographical distance often left grandparents without the capacity to process or cope with the diagnosis, which in turn impeded their ability to communicate with the grandchild with a hearing impairment, and thus impeded their ability to form a meaningful relationship. Geographical proximity enables grandparents to familiarize themselves with the child's environment and learn how to communicate with him or her.

Long distances are one of the main obstacles to forming and maintaining ongoing intergenerational relationships. Notably however, in the last decade, technological developments have changed this situation by offering various solutions such as internet text and face-to-face communications, which enable grandparents and children to conduct long and meaningful conversations on a routine basis. These changes and their impact on the family relationships have not yet been thoroughly examined in the literature.

3.10 Personal Growth Among Grandparents of a Child with a Disability

The birth of a grandchild with typical development is generally regarded as an unmitigated blessing (Findler et al. 2013). In contrast, the birth of a grandchild with a disability tends to be depicted as bleak and unfortunate. For many years, until the late 1980s, a child's disability was seen as having significant exclusive negative repercussions on all family members—who often experienced chronic grieving, suffering, misfortune, ongoing crisis, depression, stress, and existential distress (Blacher 1984; Crnic et al. 1983; Olshanksy 1962; Seligman and Darling 1989; Turnbull and Turnbull 1990; Wolfensberger and Menolascino 1970). However, it became increasingly evident that childhood disability was experienced and addressed differently in different families; some families would cope and adapt and others felt overwhelmed and burdened. This difference raised many questions about adaptation, and led researchers to examine the factors that contribute to or inhibit adaptation to childhood disability. Thus, many dimensions of adaptation were examined, including psychological adaptation (e.g., Florian and Findler 2001); marital adaptation (e.g., Kersh et al. 2006; Suarez and Baker 1997); physical adaptation (e.g., Oelofsen and Richardson 2006); and parental functioning (Baker and Heller 1996).

Whereas many researchers continued discussing the negative aspects of the crisis related to childhood disability and the factors that could facilitate adaptation (Florian and Findler 2001; Wallander et al. 1989), the first signs of the new, more positive and hopeful approach, began to appear in books written by parents of a child with a disability, who described a different picture of parenting than the one painted in the professional literature. While the picture painted by the parents did contain the elements of hardship and pain, it also revealed a sense of distinctiveness, triumph, and strength. Parents spoke of the gap between their personal experiences and the messages they received from healthcare professionals and society as a whole. Although this group of writers was small, their voices carried a new message which was impossible to ignore. Parents described emotional and spiritual development, improvement in marital relations, a new view of the world, wonder at the reactions of siblings without a disability, and a change in the family dynamics (Dougan et al. 1979; Good et al. 1985; Turnbull and Turnbull 1990). Similar testimonies were reported in qualitative studies which listed a range of insights regarding new-found emotions, the development of intimate relationships, and other positive changes that took place after the birth of a child with a disability (e.g., Scorgie et al. 1996; Stainton and Besser 1998).

There is no doubt that families of a child with a disability are faced with a formidable challenge. However, it would appear that despite the difficulties, stress, and hardship, many families adapt to the circumstances and live rich full lives replete with positive benefits, new insights, and growth (Findler and Vardi 2009; Hastings and Taunt 2002; Konrad 2006). As a result of this understanding, the literature began to present a fuller picture of families' experience of disability. Studies that adopted this new, more positive, approach towards understanding the experiences of grandparents of a child with a disability, sought to both remedy the nearly exclusive literary focus on the negative aspects of grandparenting a child with a disability (i.e. stress and burden), as well as to explore the common assumption that the absence of a disability results in a completely positive experience of grandparenthood (Findler 2014). For example, Findler (2014) found that grandparents of a child with a disability and grandparents of children without a disability reported the same degree of positive responses to grandparenthood, with the grandparents of children without a disability reporting more negative affect. Some of the participants in the study whose grandchildren did not have a disability admitted candidly that although their new role in the family was a source of love and joy, it was also quite demanding. According to one grandmother:

> *In contrast to the whole romantic thing, it's another stage in life that requires work. To tell the truth...it's not an easy job. I feel it's a burden, work, and giving.*

In contrast, instead of focusing on the negativity, demands, and burden, grandparents of a child with a disability often strove to convey optimism and strength, and focused more on mobilizing to help their children and grandchildren.

Personal growth is defined in the literature as positive changes and finding meaning in the face of crisis or existential distress (Tedeschi and Calhoun 1995). Growth is a process associated with stressful situations and/or events which lead individuals to fundamentally doubt their view of themselves and of the world; in such situations of stress, individuals' typical coping mechanisms are no longer effective or appropriate. Growth that emerges from such a context may be manifested in a number of ways including a new appreciation of life, an enhanced sense of strength and power, improved interpersonal relationships, changed priorities, spiritual development, or the discovery of new meaning and purpose in life. Various terms and definitions are used in the literature to describe these changes, such as stress-related growth (Park et al. 1996), posttraumatic growth (Tedeschi and Calhoun 2004), benefit-findings (McMillen and Cook 2003), and thriving and adversity growth (Linley and Joseph 2004).

According to Tedeschi and Calhoun (1995), while crisis and trauma may generate negative responses such as depression, helplessness, and distress, it may also be construed as a challenge which can lead to positive changes. Specifically, as a result of the cognitive and emotional process following a crisis, sometimes the trauma is perceived as having positive meaning in the present or for the future. Such a change in perspective helps individuals understand themselves and the world in a new way, and may lead to positive changes in behavior and functioning. Unexpectedly, those who undergo crisis often regard themselves as smarter, more mature, and more blessed following, and perhaps even due to their experience. A person's understanding of a crisis and the meaning he or she attributes to it have a crucial effect on the manner in which they cope with the event and its consequences (Janoff-Bulman 1992; Lazarus and Folkman 1984; Schaefer and Moos 1992; Taylor 1983).

The newly gained positivity and growth identified by parents of a child with a disability led researchers to examine the potential positive implications on additional family members, including siblings (e.g., Findler and Vardi 2009) and grandparents (e.g. Findler 2014; Findler et al. 2014; Schilmoeller and Baranowski 1998; Woodbridge et al. 2011).

Studies conducted since the mid 1990s occasionally found evidence that the difficulty and pain reported by grandparents following the birth of a child with a disability was accompanied by recognition of favorable aspects of themselves and their family members. Schilmoeller and Baranowski (1998), for example, described how over time, negative feelings were replaced with positive emotions such as acceptance, security, blessing, gratitude, strength, and vitality. Similarly, Woodbridge et al. (2011) found that grandparents of a child with a disability, for whom this was not their first grandchild, felt that the experience of grandparenting a child with a disability forced them to reexamine their values and priorities, as well as their identity as grandparents. They felt proud of the key role they played in caring for the child and of the flexibility they displayed in their willingness and ability to move from one identity to the other. Grandparents also reported taking pride in their child's strength and coping mechanisms, the grandchild's achievements, and in the unconditional love and devotion displayed by their child's spouse towards their grandchild (Woodbridge et al. 2009). Nonetheless, these reports were largely anecdotal, and did not paint a complete picture of the potential positive aspects of having a grandchild with a disability.

Tedeschi and Calhoun (2004) and Calhoun and Tedeschi (2006) further developed a model of posttraumatic growth, categorizing positive outcomes of crisis in broad domains: changes in self-perception: strength and new possibilities; changes in interpersonal relations; and changes in life philosophy: priority, appreciation, and spirituality. To further examine the experience of grandparents of a child with a disability and the potential positive implications of such a circumstance, Findler (2009) conducted a qualitative study that identified the major themes of growth among grandparents in accordance with this model.

Findler's (2009) study, which examined 38 grandparents of children with an intellectual disability and 19 grandparents of children with typical development, found that participants in both groups reported growth; in the wake of grandparenthood, all of them had feelings they had never had before, an intensity of emotion that was not produced by other contexts in their lives. Positive outcomes ranged from a new sensation of joy and happiness to physical changes and a sense of renewed energy. As one grandmother stated:

> *The pleasure is unbelievable. It does something incredible from a lot of perspectives, particularly the emotional. It opens new channels. I think there's even something hormonal in the story.*

Another grandmother remarked:

> *It's everything in my life. I'm ecstatic that I'm a grandmother. It's the best time of my life.*

Grandparenthood also allowed these individuals an opportunity to reflect on their lives and compare their functioning as parents with their role as grandparent. This comparison shed light on their personal development, greater maturity, and the new skills they had acquired since raising their own children. In the words of one grandmother:

It activates systems I didn't have with my children. There's no question it's something different...Here, with the grandchildren you're much more grown up, much more mature in a lot of ways. You're more available, you don't get angry any more. Here anything is possible. Your whole attitude comes from an entirely different place. It's different.

The grandparents felt their new role revealed aspects of their personality that had not been apparent in earlier years and in previous roles. As one grandmother stated:

Anyone who knows me wouldn't say I'm soft. I was always the strong one. I discovered my sensitivity and sentimentality. I didn't know how sensitive I was. They drew my soft underbelly out of me. It's very moving.

Although both grandparents of a child with a disability and grandparents of a child without a disability reported growth, the growth was similar in some dimensions and different in others: Among the grandparents of children with typical development, growth was expressed in feelings of unadulterated pride, new abilities, and great pleasure in the grandchild's achievements. Among the grandparents of a child with a disability, growth was generally mixed with feelings of hardship and pain. Thus, unlike anticipated normative events in the life of the family, the birth of a child with a disability is often a shock that may generate the type of experience described in the literature as posttraumatic or stress-related growth. The grandparents' growth manifested itself in the domains defined by Tedeschi and Calhoun (2004): A change in self-perception, interpersonal relationships, and change in life philosophy.

Grandparents experienced an increased sense of personal strength becuase the birth of the grandchild with a disability, and his or her presence in their lives, enabled them to learn about their own capacities. They discovered in themselves qualities such as sensitivity, patience, and empathy, along with wisdom and the ability to find information and suggest effective solutions. According to one of the grandmothers:

I knew before that I was very open and tolerant of people who are different, but I got confirmation of it. I discovered a depth of feeling in myself that I pretty much denied before.

Grandparents found themselves learning the new skills needed for the child with a disability and his or her family, as well as developing a special sensitivity which was needed in the times when stress and emotions ran high and any word could easily be misunderstood and hurt the child or the parents. A significant change in affect was also experienced by grandfathers, who reported that although throughout their lives they had restrained their feelings both at work and at home, the birth of the grandchild with a disability sobered them up and they became deluged with emotions which they no longer hid from those close to them.

Alongside this new-found sensitivity, grandparents are often required to commit themselves to the family of the child with a disability and lend practical assistance. Their response to the new needs with which the family is confronted reveals an altruism of which the grandparents are quite proud. In the words of one grandmother:

I learned that I know how to give, that I'm very strong, that I'm willing to give up everything in return for being able to offer support, for being able to help overcome the crisis.

More meaningful interpersonal relationships, another domain of growth, also emerged from grandparents' reports. This change was manifest in the enhancement of marital relations between the couple (the two grandparents), who, after many years together, began to develop a new closeness. As one grandmother remarked:

I think becoming grandparents brought us together in a special way that's new and different and very strong. Today we share experiences that give us both a lot of joy, and that creates a strong bond. My husband, who didn't share at all in raising our children, now helps a great deal and is very involved because he's compensating himself for the time he didn't give the children. It makes me very happy. I really enjoy watching him in these situations that didn't happen before. He's gentler. I'm finding sides in him I never knew before. He's opened up.

Grandfathers also expressed renewed appreciation of their wives. As one grandfather put it:

I've learned that my wife has an infinite capacity to give. She gave of herself before too, it's just greater now. I always admired her, she's always been special, but now she's twice as much the object of my admiration.

In addition, the grandparents enjoyed and felt enriched by a new level and type of dialogue with their children. They reported a two-fold benefit in terms of the pleasure and reward they got from their grandchildren along with closer relationships with their own children. The tight bond with their children led to a pattern of interpersonal relations that was significant and profound, and helped to mend past misunderstandings as well. The grandparents felt that they began to earn their children's appreciation and gratitude for their help and support. Nearly 90 % of the grandparents in Anderson's report (2010a) felt that the experience of facing their grandchild's situation together had brought them and their adult child closer. Many expressed pride in their child's strength and commitment as he or she faced raising a child with a disability. In the words of a Grandmother:

We're there in 10 minutes whenever she asks. It mellowed the relationship between us. She suddenly saw what I'm willing to do for her. Paradoxically, the child brought us closer together. It's like a gift in the midst of all the hardship.

Additionally, grandparents learned to appreciate their children more. Specifically, they reported being impressed by their children's parenting skills and the way they in which they had suddenly gone from being dependent to being independent mothers and fathers with impressive values and priorities from which the grandparents themselves could learn. Before their very eyes, their "spoiled" child had become a devoted parent, investing all of his or her effort in the child. According to one of the grandfathers:

I don't have words to describe it, I really don't. What parents he (the grandchild) has. That's probably the reason such incredible things are happening with the child.

Another grandfather remarked:

My daughter and her husband are amazing. They grew up to be parents and human beings, and I really think that in this sense the grandchild is a gift. He's always teaching us about ourselves.

The change in interpersonal relations was felt outside the framework of the family as well. Participants reported that since the birth of the grandchild with a disability, those social relationships that remained intact were based on trust. Grandparents began to invest in the quality of their relations with friends, a trend characterized by building deeper and more intimate relationships, and ridding their social network of superficial connections; they learned who their real friends were and made a conscious decision to surround themselves with people with whom they had meaningful relationships. Moreover, the experience of having a grandchild with a disability made them more sensitive to other children and adults in general, an attitude that also impacted their social relations positively.

In addition, acknowledgement of their hardship and vulnerability in regards to the grandchild with a disability encouraged many grandparents to seek help, with some joining support groups. Such groups typically offered them their first opportunity to share their emotions with other people in a similar situation. The ability to discuss their experience and the pain it engendered often led to greater openness and willingness to share feelings.

Grandparents of a child with a disability also reported a change in philosophy of life: priorities, appreciation, and spirituality, the third domain of growth. Specifically, grandparents of a child with a disability often undergo a crisis of values. For example, on the one hand, they belong to a society that worships physical perfection and intellectual achievements, a society in which disability or illness are perceived as a tragedy, inferiority and/or flaw (Livneh 1988). On the other hand, social norms dictate that one is expected to accept and love their children and grandchildren unconditionally. As a result of this conflict, the grandparents are forced to modify the value system in which they were raised, a system upheld by their surrounding social environment, and to learn to value different qualities (Menolascino 1968; Wolfensberger 1967). Grandparents' in Findler's (2009) study found themselves reevaluating attitudes they had always taken for granted. This change was expressed, for example, in celebrating a small improvement as achievement and/or relating differently to physical appearance. Woodbridge et al. (2009) similarly report that grandparents of a child with a disability took great pride in their grandchild's achievements, feeling that every small step was beyond all expectations.

The change in philosophy is also expressed in more clearly defined life goals, which are the products of an internal cognitive process that takes place in the wake of a negative event. Paradoxically, in order for positive changes to occur, the negative event must be sufficiently unsettling to alter people's perspective of themselves or of the world. As McMillen and Fisher (1998) mention, research suggests that often people with the highest exposure to the negative event are the ones most likely to perceive benefit (McMillen et al. 1997; Park et al. 1996; Tedeschi and Calhoun 1996). In the words of one grandfather:

The child taught me that you have to invest more and believe more. Above all, you have to believe. I was not a believer.

Some grandparents felt new dimensions of spirituality or closeness to God as expressed by a grandmother:

...I have a talk with GOD every morning, and I thank Him, something that I had never done before. With time, I see things differently... I see that I have to take advantage of every day in my life, not to dwell in the past or the future, and I'm very much concerned with the issue of health. One cannot always implement this, but every day is an extra gift...

The gap between the qualitative studies that highlight the positive experiences of families with a child with a disability and the earlier quantitative studies that cast a shadow on this experience indicated that a different type of "lighting" was required to discern the positive aspects in family life. Consequently, new quantitative research aimed at exploring the positive implications of harsh life events began to appear in the literature. Based on initial research findings, instruments were devised by King and Patterson (2000), Scorgie et al. (2004), and Stainton and Besser (1998), to measure growth from adversity. Some of these measures were used to examine the experiences of parents of a child with a disability.

Two recent quantitative studies investigated, for the first time, the positive repercussions and sense of growth among grandparents of a child with an intellectual disability (Findler 2014) and of grandparents of a child diagnosed with cancer (Findler et al. 2014). In the first study, 94 grandparents of a child with an intellectual disability were compared with 105 grandparents of a child with typical development to identify similarities and differences between the groups. The Post Traumatic Growth model suggested by Schaefer and Moos (1992) was used to examine variables that might influence perceptions of the crisis and contribute to positive outcomes. The variables that were examined included: event-related factors, represented by the presence of a grandchild with a disability; personal traits, examined through self-differentiation, perception of four dimensions of grandparenthood (emotional, symbolic, cognitive, and behavioral), demographic characteristics such as age and gender; and environmental factors, represented by family cohesion and flexibility and social support. The coping resources included in the original model of Schaefer and Moos (1992) were not examined in the study.

The findings revealed similar responses amongst both groups of grandparents. Specifically, a relatively high level of growth as well as similar internal and external contributors to growth were found among all the participants. The differences between the two groups were not associated with the presence or absence of a disability, but rather with demographic characteristics: differences were found between men and women, between older and younger grandparents, and between those in better and poorer health. Not surprisingly, woman, who are typically more invested in their family roles and regard them as a form of self-fulfillment, reported higher personal growth than men, as did grandparents who were younger and in better health. As advanced age and poorer health may cause discomfort, illness, or physical restrictions, such grandparents can be expected to find it harder to invest the effort required for intensive involvement or interactions with their grandchildren.

The symbolic dimension of grandparenthood contributed to personal growth in both groups of grandparents in the study. This dimension relates to the pleasure and satisfaction derived from the role as compared with the role of parent, or in the sense of immortality or continuity it may provide (Neugarten and Weinstein 1964). The respondents felt that as grandparents they were compensating for what they had missed out on as parents, and felt that grandparenthood gave them the opportunity to improve their relationships with their own children. Moreover, grandparenthood gave them the opportunity to express their vitality and capabilities, and contribute to the family, all of which afforded them a sense of personal growth and accomplishment.

Personal growth was also experienced by grandparents who reported less negative affect associated with the role of grandparent. This connection is consistent with the findings of other studies that adopted the approach of positive psychology (e.g., Fredrickson 2005). Negative emotions can have devastating effects and amongst other things, may be expressed in depression and rage. While such negative responses may arise in any interaction with a grandchild, the less frequently they occur and the better the individual's emotional state is, the more growth they experience from their role as grandparent. Taking an active part in expanding the child's knowledge affords grandparents an appreciation of their importance to the family and the special role they play in the child's life; such feelings contribute to a sense of personal growth. The more the grandparents were involved in educating and enriching their grandchild, the more growth they reported.

The external resource of family cohesion, i.e. the degree of emotional connect or disconnect among family members (Olson et al. 1983), also contributed to a stronger sense of growth among participants in the study (Findler 2014). A high level of family cohesion facilitates harmonious intergenerational relationships and the ability to derive pleasure and satisfaction from being a grandparent. Those reporting a high level of cohesion felt that their family experienced close emotional ties, clearly defined boundaries, interest in each other's lives, and good communications, all of which enabled the expression of both positive and negative feelings. As family cohesion affects the individual functioning as well as the family as a whole (Moos and Moos 1976; Russel 1979), it is not surprising that it was found to predict the personal growth of grandparents.

The second study referred to above (Findler et al. 2014) compared 56 grandparents of a child who survived cancer with 60 grandparents of healthy children. It was found that within two to three years after the grandchild's recovery, the grandparents had resumed their routine and reported a quality of life similar to that of the grandparents of healthy children. However, the difficult period the family had undergone and the support grandparents had offered during that time took a toll on the grandparents' health. Yet despite having to pay this price, grandparents reported higher personal growth than the comparison group. Their growth was reflected in all three domains: greater appreciation of themselves, improvement in interpersonal relations and in the importance they attributed to them, and a change in their worldview and philosophy of life. The complex picture which shows greater growth among the grandparents of a child who recovered from cancer, reveals the uniqueness of personal growth namely, growth is a reflection of change.

This contention is further supported by the differences that emerged between the pattern of contributions of internal resources to the personal growth and quality of life of these grandparents. While a high level of coherence contributed to the quality of life of grandparents, a low level of this resource contributed to growth. According to Antonovsky (1987), people with a strong sense of coherence perceive events in their lives as less threatening, have faith in their ability to cope with challenges, and adapt to difficult situations more easily. Hence, when faced with a dramatic life crisis, grandparents with a high level of this trait could call on this crucial resource. Despite the circumstances, they believed their world to be comprehensible, manageable, and predictable, and were thus generally able to maintain balance and overcome the crisis or stress with the help of their personal resources. As a result, they displayed better adaptation and succeeded in maintaining their quality of life and normal routine. In contrast, grandparents with limited internal resources found themselves to be lacking control and felt a high level of uncertainty in their world which they felt to be chaotic. The crisis disrupted their lives to the extent that it compelled them to change. Seeking out new sources of strength and coping, they discovered features and capacities within themselves that they had been previously unaware of; in other words, they experienced growth (Findler et al. 2014).

All the grandparents in these two studies showed similar degrees of joy and happiness in their roles, along with similar degrees of new-found softness, patience, readiness, and commitment. In the interpersonal realm as well, grandparents expressed renewed appreciation for their spouses, children, and grandchildren. These studies reinforce that grandparenthood can welcome an opportunity to reevaluate and improve relationships, and to compensate for what grandparents had lacked or missed out on in the past. However, grandparents of a child with an intellectual disability or life-threatening illness were distinct from grandparents of children with typical development in terms of the content and intensity of the experiences they described. For grandparents of a child with a disability, the joy and happiness are mixed with pain, concern, and sorrow. In contrast to the similarities found in the personal and interpersonal dimensions, a change in the third domain of growth, philosophy of life, was seen by grandparents of a child with a disability or illness. Despite their years and experience, the presence of this grandchild caused a major disruption that led to a reexamination of former priorities, worldview, and attitudes, which resulted in a modification of their philosophy of life, a hallmark of growth.

Grandmothers and grandfathers are an important part of the support system of their families, particularly when a grandchild has a disability. Until now, most of the literature focused on these grandparents' roles and contributions to the nuclear family (i.e. to their children and grandchildren). This chapter illuminated the unique experiences of the grandparents themselves. With all of the complexity and vulnerability in intergenerational relationships, grandparents who feel valued, feel that they have a unique role, and feel like they can contribute to all that is happening in the family, also experience vitality, meaning in their lives, and even growth. In sum, without understanding the process that grandparents go through, the implications of having a grandchild with a disability on their lives, and the various meanings of intergenerational connections in this context, it would not be possible to get the best from this unique asset of the family.

References

Anderson, C. (2010a). *Grandparents of children with ASD: Part 1*. Baltimore, MD: Kennedy Krieger Institute. Retrieved from: http://www.iancommunity.org/cs/ian_research_reports/ian_research_report_apr_2010

Anderson, C. (2010b). *Grandparents of children with ASD: Part 2*. Baltimore, MD: Kennedy Krieger Institute. Retrieved from: http://www.iancommunity.org/cs/ianresearch_reports/ian_research_report_apr_2010_2

Antonovsky, A. (1987). *Unraveling the mystery of health: How people manage stress and stay well*. San Francisco, CA: Jossey-Bass.

Baker, B. L., & Heller, T. L. (1996). Preschool children with externalizing behaviors: Experience of fathers and mothers. *Journal of Abnormal Child Psychology, 24*, 513–532.

Bates, J. S. (2009). Generative grandfathering: A conceptual framework for nurturing grandchildren. *Marriage and Family Review, 45*(331–352), 352.

Bengtson, V. L., & Mangen, D. J. (1988). Family intergenerational solidarity revisited: Suggestions for future management. In D. J. Mangen, V. L. Bengtson, & P. H. Landry (Eds.), *Measurement of intergenerational relations* (pp. 222–238). Thousand Oaks, CA: Sage Publications Inc.

Bengtson, V. L., & Roberts, R. E. L. (1991). Intergenerational solidarity in aging families: An example of formal theory construction. *Journal of Marriage and the Family, 53*, 856–870.

Bernier, J. C. (1990). Parental adjustment to a disabled child: A family-system perspective. *Families in Society, 71*, 589–596.

Berns, J. H. (1980). Grandparents of handicapped children. *Social Work, 25*, 238–239.

Blacher, J. (1984). Sequential stages of parental adjustment to the birth of a child with handicaps: Fact or artifact? *Mental Retardation, 22*, 55–68.

Bowen, M. (1978). *Family therapy in clinical practice*. Lanham, MD: Jason Aronson.

Burns, C. E., & Madian, N. (1992). Experiences with a support group for grandparents of children with disabilities. *Pediatric Nursing, 18*, 17–21.

Calhoun, L. G., & Tedeschi, R. G. (2006). The foundations of posttraumatic growth: An expanded framework. In L.G. Calhoun, & R.G. Tedeschi (Eds.), *Handbook of posttraumatic growth: Research & practice*. (pp.1–23) Mahwah, NJ: Lawrence Erlbaum Associates Publishers.

Crnic, K. A., Friedrich, W. N., & Greenberg, M. T. (1983). Adaptation of families with mentally retarded children: A model of stress, coping, and family ecology. *American Journal of Mental Deficiency, 88*, 125–138.

Dougan, T., Isbell, L., & Vyas, P. (1979). *We have been there*. Salt Lake City, UT: Dougan, Isbell and Vyas Associates.

Drew, L. M., Richard, M. H., & Smith, P. K. (1998). Grandparenting and its relationship to parenting. *Clinical Child Psychology and Psychiatry, 3*, 465–480.

Findler, L. (2000). The role of grandparents in the social support system of mothers of children with a physical disability. *Families in Society: The Journal of Contemporary human services, 81*, 370–381.

Findler, L. (2009). *The experience of grandparenthood among grandparents of children with/without an intellectual disability: The contribution of self-differentiation, social support and the perception of grandparenthood to personal growth*. Submitted to Shalem fund for the development of services of for people with intellectual disabilities in the local councils in Israel.

Findler, L. (2014). The experience of stress and personal growth among grandparents of children with and without intellectual disabilities. *Intellectual and Developmental Disabilities, 52*, 32–48.
Findler, L., & Vardi, A. (2009). Psychological growth among siblings of children with and without intellectual disabilities. *Intellectual and Developmental Disabilities, 47*, 1–12.
Findler, L., Dayan-Sharabi, M., & Yaniv, I. (2014). The overlooked side of the experience: Personal growth and quality of life among grandparents of children who survived cancer. *Journal of Family Social Work, 17*, 418–437.
Findler, L., Taubman-Ben-Ari, O., Nuttman-Shwartz, O., & Lazar, R. (2013). Construction and validation of the multidimensional experience of grandparenthood set of inventories. *Social Work Research, 37*, 237–253.
Fischer, L. R., & Silverman, J. (1982). *Grandmothering as a "tenuous" role relationship*. Paper presented at the National Council on Family Relations, Portland, OR.
Florian, V., & Findler, L. (2001). Mental health and marital adaptation among mothers of children with cerebral palsy. *American Journal of Orthopsychiatry, 71*, 358–367.
Fredrickson, B. (2005). Positive emotions. In C. R. Snyder & S. J. Lopez (Eds.), *Handbook of positive psychology* (pp. 120–134). New York, NY: University Press.
Gallagher, P. A., Kresak, K., & Rhodes, C. A. (2010). Perceived needs of grandmothers of children with disabilities. *Topics in Early Childhood Special Education, 30*, 56–64.
Gardner, J. E., Scherman, A., Mobley, D., Brown, P., & Schutter, M. (1994). Grandparents' beliefs regarding their role and relationship with special needs grandchildren. *Education and Treatment of Children, 17*, 185–196.
George, J. D. (1988). Therapeutic intervention for grandparents and extended family of children with developmental delays. *Mental Retardation, 26*, 369–375.
Good, J. D., Reis, J. G., & Henderson, J. (1985). *A special kind of parenting: Meeting the needs of handicapped children*. Chicago, IL: La Leche League International.
Green, S. E. (2001). Grandma's hands: Parental perceptions of the importance of grandparents as secondary caregivers in families with disabilities. *International Journal of Aging and Human Development, 53*, 11–33.
Hall, O. C. (2004). A double concern: Grandparents' experiences when a small grandchild is critically ill. *Journal of Pediatric Nursing, 19*, 61–69.
Hastings, R. P., & Taunt, H. M. (2002). Positive perceptions in families of children with developmental disabilities. *American Journal of Mental Retardation, 107*, 116–127.
Hillman, J. (2007). Grandparents of children with autism: A review with recommendations for education, practice, and policy. *Educational Gerontology, 33*, 513–527.
Hugger, L. (2009). Mourning the loss of the idealized child. *Journal of Infant, Child and Adolescent Psychotherapy, 8*, 124–136.
Janoff-Bulman, R. (1992). *Shattered assumptions: Towards a new psychology of trauma*. New York, NY: Free Press.
Johnson, C. L. (1998). Effects of adult children's divorce on grandparenthood. In M. E. Szinovacz (Ed.), *Handbook of grandparenthood* (pp. 184–199). Westport, CT: Greenwood Press.
Katz, S., & Kessel, L. (2002). Grandparents of children with developmental disabilities: Perceptions, beliefs, and involvement in their care. *Issues in Comprehensive Pediatric Nursing, 25*, 113–128.
Kazak, A. E., & Christakis, D. A. (1994). Caregiving issues in families of children with chronic medical conditions. In E. Kahana, D. E. Biegel, & M. L. Wykle (Eds.), *Family caregiving across the lifespan* (pp. 331–356). Thousands Oaks, CA: Sage Publications.
Kersh, J., Hedvat, T. T., Hauser-Cram, P., & Warfield, M. E. (2006). The contribution of marital quality to the well-being of parents of children with developmental disabilities. *Journal of Intellectual Disability Research, 50*, 883–893.
King, L. A., & Patterson, C. (2000). Reconstructing life goals after the birth of a child with down syndrome: Finding happiness and growing. *International Journal of Rehabilitation and Health, 5*, 17–30.
Kivnick, H. Q. (1982). *The meaning of grandparenthood: Research in clinical psychology: 3*. Ann Arbor, MI: UMI Research Press.

Konrad, S. C. (2006). Posttraumatic growth in mothers of children with acquired disabilities. *Journal of Loss and Trauma, 11*, 101–113.

Lazarus, R. S., & Folkman, S. (1984). *Stress, appraisal and coping*. New York, NY: Springer Publishing.

Lee, M., & Gardner, J. E. (2010). Grandparents' involvement and support in families with children with disabilities. *Educational Gerontology, 36*, 467–499.

Linley, P. A., & Joseph, S. (2004). Positive change following trauma and adversity: A review. *Journal of Traumatic Stress, 17*, 11–21.

Livneh, H. (1988). A dimensional perspective on the origin of negative attitude towards persons with disabilities. In H. E. Yuker (Ed.), *Attitudes toward persons with disabilities* (pp. 35–46). New York, NY: Springer.

Margetts, J. K., Couteur, A. L., & Croom, S. (2006). Families in a state of flux: The experience of grandparents in autism spectrum disorder. *Child: Care, Health and Development, 32*, 565–574.

McCubbin, H. I., & Patterson, J. M. (1983). The family stress process: The double ABCX model of family adjustment and adaptation. *Marriage and Family Review, 6*, 7–37.

McMillen, J. C., & Cook, C. L. (2003). The positive by-products of spinal cord injury and their correlates. *Rehabilitation Psychology, 48*, 77–85.

McMillen, J. C., & Fisher, R. H. (1998). The perceived benefit scales: Measuring perceived positive life changes following negative life events. *Social Work Research, 22*, 173–187.

McMillen, J. C., Smith, E. M., & Fisher, R. H. (1997). Perceived benefit and mental health after three types of disaster. *Journal of Consulting and Clinical Psychology, 65*, 733–739.

Menolascino, F. J. (1968). Parents of the mentally retarded: An operational approach to diagnosis and management. *Journal of the American Academy of Child Psychiatry, 7*, 589–602.

Miller, E., Buys, L., & Woodbridge, S. (2012). Impact of disability on families: Grandparents' perspectives. *Journal of Intellectual Disability Research, 56*, 102–110.

Mirfin-Veitch, B., Bray, A., & Watson, M. (1996). "They really do care": Grandparents as informal support sources for families of children with disabilities. *New Zealand Journal of Disability Studies, 2*, 136–148.

Mirfin-Veitch, B., Bray, A., & Watson, M. (1997). "We're just that sort of family": Intergenerational relationships in families including children with disabilities. *Family Relations, 46*, 305–311.

Mitchell, W. (2008). The role played by grandparents in family support and learning: Considerations for mainstream and special schools. *Support for learning, 23*, 126–135.

Moos, R. H., & Moos, B. S. (1976). A typology of family social environments. *Family Process, 15*, 357–371.

Moules, N. J., McCaffrey, G., Laing, C. M., Tapp, D. M., & Strother, D. (2012). Grandparents' experiences of childhood cancer, part 2: The need for support. *Journal of Pediatric Oncology Nursing, 29*, 133–140.

Neugarten, B. L., & Weinstein, K. K. (1964). The changing American grandparent. *Journal of Marriage and the Family, 26*, 199–204.

Nybo, W. L., Scherman, A., & Freeman, P. L. (1998). Grandparents' role in family systems with a deaf child: An exploratory study. *American Annals of the Deaf, 143*, 260–267.

Oelofsen, N., & Richardson, P. (2006). Sense of coherence and parenting stress in mothers and fathers of preschool children with developmental disability. *Journal of Intellectual and Developmental Disability, 31*, 1–12.

Olshanksy, S. (1962). Chronic sorrow: A response to having a mentally defective child. *Social Case Work, 43*, 190–193.

Olson, D. H., Russell, C. S., & Sprenkle, D. H. (1983). Circumplex model of marital and family systems: VI. Theoretical update. *Family Process, 22*, 69–83.

Park, C. L., Cohen, L. H., & Murch, R. L. (1996). Assessment and prediction of stress-related growth. *Journal of Personality, 64*, 71–106.

Riesz, E. D. (2004). Loss and transitions: A 30-year perspective on life with a child who has down syndrome. *Journal of Loss and Trauma, 9*, 371–382.

Rossi, A. S., & Rossi, P. H. (1990). *Of human bonding: Parent-child relations across the life course*. Hawthorne, NY: Aldine de Gruyter.

Russel, C. S. (1979). Circumplex model of marital and family systems: III. Empirical evaluation with families. *Family Process, 18*, 29–45.

Schaefer, J. A., & Moos, G. H. (1992). Life crises and personal growth. In B. N. Carpenter (Ed.), *Personal coping: Theory, research and application* (pp. 149–170). Westport, CT: Praeger Publishers.

Scherman, A., Gardner, J. E., Brown, P., & Schutter, M. (1995). Grandparents' adjustment to grandchildren with disabilities. *Educational Gerontology, 21*, 261–273.

Schilmoeller, G., & Baranowski, M. (1998). Intergenerational support in families with disabilities: Grandparents' perspectives. *Families in Society: The Journal of Contemporary Social Services, 79*, 465–476.

Scorgie, K., Wilgosh, L., & McDonald, L. (1996). A qualitative study of managing life when a child has a disability. *Developmental Disabilities Bulletin, 24*, 68–90.

Scorgie, K., Wilgosh, L., & Sobsey, D. (2004). The experience of transformation in parents of children with disabilities: Theoretical Considerations. *Developmental Disabilities Bulletin, 32*, 84–110.

Seligman, M. (1991). Grandparents of disabled grandchildren: Hopes, fears, and adaptation. *Families in Society, 72*, 147–152.

Seligman, M., & Darling, R. B. (1989). *Ordinary families, special children: A systems approach to childhood disability*. New York, NY: The Guilford Press.

Seligman, M., Goodwin, G., Paschal, K., Applegate, A., & Lehman, L. (1997). Grandparents of children with disabilities: Perceived levels of support. *Education and Training in Mental Retardation and Developmental Disabilities, 32*, 293–303.

Shaw, S. L. (2005). Grandparent Involvement in the communication development of children who are deafblind. *Educational Gerontology, 31*, 51–71.

Stainton, T., & Besser, H. (1998). The positive impact of children with an intellectual disability on the family. *Journal of Intellectual and Developmental Disability, 23*, 57–70.

Suarez, L. M., & Baker, B. L. (1997). Child externalizing behavior and parents' stress: The role of social support. *Family Relations, 46*, 373–381.

Sullivan, A., Winograd, G., Verkuilen, J., & Fish, M. C. (2012). Children on the autism spectrum: Grandmother involvement and family functioning. *Journal of Applied Research in Intellectual Disabilities, 25*, 484–494.

Taylor, S. E. (1983). Adjustment to threatening events: A theory of cognitive adaptation. *American Psychologist, 38*, 1161–1173.

Tedeschi, R. G., & Calhoun, L. G. (1995). *Trauma and transformation: Growing in the aftermath of suffering*. Thousand Oaks, CA: Sage Publications.

Tedeschi, R. G., & Calhoun, L. G. (1996). The posttraumatic growth inventory: Measuring the positive legacy of trauma. *Journal of Traumatic Stress, 9*, 455–471.

Tedeschi, R. G., & Calhoun, L. G. (2004). Posttraumatic growth: Conceptual foundations and empirical evidence. *Psychological Inquiry, 15*, 1–18.

Thomas, J. L. (1986). Gender differences in satisfaction with grandparenting. *Psychology and Aging, 1*, 215–219.

Trute, B. (2003). Grandparents of children with developmental disabilities: Intergenerational support and family well-being. *Families in Society: The Journal of Contemporary Social Services, 84*, 119–126.

Turnbull, A. P., & Turnbull, H. R. (1990). *Families, professionals, and exceptionality: A special partnership*. Columbus, OH: Merrill Publishing Company.

Vadasy, P. F. (1987). Grandparents of children with special needs: Supports especially for grandparents. *Children's Health Care, 16*, 21–23.

Wallander, J. L., Pitt, L. C., & Mellins, C. A. (1990). Child functional independence and maternal psychosocial stress as risk factors threatening adaptation in mothers of physically or sensorially handicapped children. *Journal of Consulting and Clinical Psychology, 58*, 818–824.

Wallander, J. L., Varni, J. W., Babani, L., Banis, H. T., & Wilcox, K. T. (1989). Family resources as resistance factors for psychological maladjustment in chronically ill and handicapped children. *Journal of Pediatric Psychology, 14*, 157–173.

Whittingham, K., Wee, D., Sanders, M. R., & Boyd, R. (2013). Sorrow, coping and resiliency: Parents of children with cerebral palsy share their experiences. *Disability and Rehabilitation: An International, Multidisciplinary Journal, 35*, 1447–1452.

Wikler, L., Wasow, M., & Hatfield, E. (1981). Chronic sorrow revisited: Parent vs. professional depiction of the adjustment of parents of mentally retarded children. *American Journal of Orthopsychiatry, 51*, 63–70.

Wolfensberger, W. (1967). Counselling the parents of the retarded. In A. A. Baumeisten (Ed.), *Mental reatardation: Appraisal, education, and rehabilitation* (pp. 329–400). Chicago, LA: Aldine Publishing Company.

Wolfensberger, W., & Menolascino, F. J. (1970). A theoretical framework for the management of parents of the mentally retarded. In F. J. Menolascino (Ed.), *Psychiatric approaches to mental retardation* (pp. 475–493). New York, NY: Basic Books.

Woodbridge, S., Buys, L., & Miller, E. (2009). Grandparenting a child with a disability: An emotional rollercoaster. *Australasian Journal on Ageing, 28*, 37–40.

Woodbridge, S., Buys, L., & Miller, E. (2011). 'My grandchild has a disability': Impact on grandparenting identity, roles and relationships. *Journal on Ageing Studies, 25*, 355–363.

Chapter 4
Grandparents of Children with Disabilities—The Parents' Perspective

(Grand) Parents Are Forever Parents

Liora Findler

Abstract This chapter examines the role of the grandparents of children with disabilities from the point of view of the parents, the middle generation. It describes the unique contribution of the grandparents to the parents' adjustment to their new reality, considering how each of the parents perceives the place of the grandfathers versus the grandmothers, and the maternal grandparents versus the paternal grandparents. The chapter relates at length to the costs and benefits of the relationship with the grandparents, examining differences between the two generations in respect to expectations, channels of communication, and the provision or non-provision of support, as well as the parents' assessment of the quality of the grandparents' involvement.

Keywords Grandparenthood · Grandchildren with a disability · Parents perspective · Intergenerational relationship · Social support · Paternal and maternal grandparents

Anticipating the birth of a child is one of the most meaningful experiences in life. It brings with it exciting promise, arousing in the parents-to-be the expectation of self-fulfillment, unconditional love and giving, and a special relationship with the growing child. In view of the intensity of this virtually universal response, the news that the child has been born with a disability often marks the start of a descent into a world where hopes are dashed and expectations belied.

> *Her first year was simply catastrophic; I felt like one of the loneliest people in the universe. From a person of a lot of doing, having a career, very active life, I was completely neglecting myself, stuck with a baby, a restless, horrible baby, and I was totally devoting myself, and at the same time, my whole family was busy with their lives, and I was so lonely, I was all alone.*

This chapter provides a review of the literature on parents of a child with a disability and their views on the role of grandparents in their families. The review will also include the voices of parents from interviews (conducted specifically for this chapter) with mothers and fathers of children with disabilities.

L. Findler and O. Taubman – Ben-Ari, *Grandparents of Children with Disabilities*,
SpringerBriefs in Well-Being and Quality of Life Research,
DOI 10.1007/978-3-319-45517-4_4

The parents of children with disabilities frequently express feelings of solitude and the sense that they are carrying a heavy burden that cannot be lightened by being shared with others. They speak of the strong impact on their financial situation, their time for themselves, and the future of the family, as well as the effect on other family members and on their relationships with them. The implications of the birth of a child with a disability on the parents have been described over the years in the literature as an extended crisis and a source of depression, stress, and existential distress (Barnett and Boyce 1995; Case-Smith 2012; Crnic et al. 1983; Florian and Findler 2001; Friedrich and Friedrich 1981; Glidden and Schoolcraft 2003; Wolfensberger and Menolascino 1970). As in the case of other life crises, the family ultimately acquires a fuller picture of the situation and settles into a routine in which most parents adjust and some even experience personal and familial growth (Finzi-Dottan et al. 2011; Larson 2010; Manor-Binyamini 2014; Resch et al. 2012).

Despite the similar demands on families of children with disabilities, the literature demonstrates growing awareness of the different ways in which individual families and parents experience this reality. Many scholars have wondered why certain families cope and adapt, while others collapse under the burden (Tak and McCubbin 2002). This question has given rise to investigations of the internal and external factors that may enhance or inhibit adaptation. One of the major resources shown to promote parental coping is social support, and particularly the support of grandparents. As a link in the generational chain, grandparents are often deeply emotionally involved and are seen to have a stake in the fate and continuity of the family, and thus parents frequently find it easier to share their feelings with them.

Many studies and reports in the literature on the tri-generational relationship in families of children with disabilities deal with the issue from the standpoint of the grandparents (Findler 2014; Gardner et al. 2004; Vadasy 1987). The current chapter examines the grandparents' place in these families from the perspective of the child's parents through a review of the literature intertwined with quotes from interviews with parents of children with disabilities.

4.1 Grandparents' Role in Families of Children with Disabilities

As an integral part of the family system, grandparents' contribution to the life of the family can affect the grandchildren's development, whether directly if they play an active role in their upbringing, or indirectly through their support for the parents (Sandler 1998). Relating to the change in the perception of grandparents' role in the modern family, Sandler (1998) relies on Kornhaber (1986), who depicts the change as a shift from the traditional manner of grandparental involvement, expressed in mutual support and close emotional ties, to the contemporary attitude in which the intergenerational relationship is also characterized by greater independence and autonomy of the nuclear family. As Sandler (1998) notes, however, in times of crisis or stress, there is a greater need for intergenerational support. When this need meets current messages of mutual independence and non-involvement, there may be confusion as to the expectations from the grandparents.

Furthermore, when parents anticipate support from the grandparents while at the same time expecting them to respect the family's autonomy, the grandparents may find themselves in a conflictual situation in which their efforts to provide assistance are construed as interference (Thomas 1990). The challenge nowadays is successful intergenerational relationships that are based on the balance between involvement and intervention.

After my father-in-law passed away, there was a kind of a renaissance in my relationship with my mother-in-law. I think that it dawned on me that I could receive her help and concern and that she would keep herself out of my business without bossing me around, so I think we've reached a good equation. (Mother of a child with a disability)

Notwithstanding the nuclear family's desire for autonomy and the tensions this may arouse, there are distinct expectations of assistance from the grandparents. Given their unique place in the fabric of the family, their relations with the other generations are complex and vary from one culture to the other, one family to the next, one period to the next, and one individual to the next. The complexity of their role is considerably more pronounced in the family of a child with a disability. As the parents are dealing with a highly sensitive and demanding reality, the need for the grandparents' support is substantially greater and its lack is more intensely felt.

From my mother, I expected much more help, more willingness to come and help and keep an eye on him, be with him. I had higher expectations; I thought it would be a lot easier for me with the grandparents. (Mother of a child with a disability)

4.2 Grandparents' Contribution to Parents' Adaptation

The grandparents' response to a grandchild with a disability may have a strong impact on their own children's sense of competence as parents. For example, when grandparents had accepted the diagnosis more quickly than the parents had, they in fact helped them shape their own attitude toward their child (Mirfin-Veitch et al. 1996). Moreover, a positive attitude on the part of the grandparents can enhance the parents' adaptation and further the development of the child (Green 2001).

The parents of children with disabilities ascribe great importance and gratitude to the support they receive from their own parents (Baranowski and Schilmoeller 1999; Bruns and Foerster 2011; Findler 2000; Green 2001; Heller et al. 2000; Lindblad et al. 2007; Seligman et al. 1997; Trute 2003).

Grandparents are meaningful, even if they don't sit and hold our hands, and give therapy sessions, they have to give that hug, the feeling that you're not alone, because even though you're a very capable person, and you keep pushing and doing, and you live a very, very,

> *sort of active life, and you can do it, you're there for your child, it is what it is, sometimes, especially those moments, the small ones, bring you to the point where you need your parents, and even if it's hard for your parents, they need to be parents, because parents are parents forever.* (Mother of a child with a disability)

Grandparents may contribute to the family's adaptation on several fronts, including emotional adaptation (mental health), the couple relationship, parental functioning, financial coping and communication among the family members. A qualitative study conducted by Green (2001) highlights the unique contribution of grandparents' support to the parents of a child with a disability. The significance of giving a grandchild with disability the same unconditional love one gives any grandchild emerges from Green's (2001) study. It was found that the grandparents' ability to take the same pride in the child with a disability that they would in any grandchild helped the parents feel part of the normative world of social and intergenerational relations and contributed to their emotional well-being.

In addition, the study found that a high level of support from the grandparents was generally accompanied by a high level of support from other sources as well, such as aunts and uncles, neighbors, or friends. However, the assistance of the grandparents was distinct in that it promoted the parents' ability to maintain a positive attitude and avoid physical exhaustion (Green 2001).

Furthermore, in families where grandparents' support was lacking, the parents reported lower emotional well-being than in those that regularly received aid from the grandparents, even though help from other sources was available (Green 2001).

> *I think this is the parents' role. As the bubble is shattered for their children, who realize that their child is not a 'regular' child, so you put aside the pain, and you go on... I talk with my friends who have "regular" children. If their parents do not provide them with physical help at least once a week, they freak out and go crazy, and they are very disappointed and there is a lot of anger. So even more, when you are in such a terrible situation, it is very, very important just to be there. If my mom, when my little one was a baby, had told me, 'get out of the house now, I don't want to see you until noon, go, go, and do something for yourself, go to sleep, whatever, I'm here with the child', then, you know, everything would have been different.* (Mother of a child with a disability)

4.3 Features of Grandparents' Support

Grandparents' support can be manifested on both the emotional and instrumental levels. Emotional support takes the form of exchanges that provide an opportunity to share thoughts, express feelings, and offer encouragement, while instrumental support includes babysitting, helping with chores, furnishing transportation, etc. (Findler 2000; Lindblad et al. 2007).

The family of a child with a disability typically has a particular need for instrumental support, such as financial assistance due to the cost of special services and equipment or help in taking the child to medical and paramedical treatments and consultations (Hillman 2007; Katz and Kessel 2002; Lee and Gardner 2010).

I really do think that the most important role of the grandparents is simply to be there, to say, what do you need, do you need three hours? Do you need a whole day, an afternoon once a week? Do you need us to come in the morning? We will come, we will be there... I think that the physical support will bring the mental well-being, because not every parent is capable of containing, coping, talking, solving things on an emotional level with their child, these are grown kids, you know, but when you are there physically and you help physically, you're helping your child mentally. (Mother of a child with a disability)

Nevertheless, studies conducted in the US, Canada and Israel all show that although the mothers of children with disabilities report receiving both instrumental and emotional support from the grandparents, they regard the emotional support as more significant (Baranowski and Schilmoeller 1999; Findler 2000; Trute 2003; Trute et al. 2008). This may be because the expectation of instrumental support in such families is more openly acknowledged than the expectation of emotional support, despite the considerable need for this form of assistance. When emotional support is received in the absence of an expressed expectation of it, it is even more conspicuous and appreciated.

My wife's mother gives a lot, sometimes she says: use me more, I'm here. She has a fixed day where she takes my son to school, basketball, lunch... Whenever we go somewhere, she is the preferred grandparent. She's a real grandmother, coddling, presents, Friday meals, they sleep over without planning in advance and she's always fine with it. Emotional support is the most essential. Since the first stage... she has been a mother figure, asking, inquiring and taking an interest. (Father of a child with a disability)

A possible explanation for the importance attributed to emotional support from grandparents is the fact that it is easier to accept instrumental help from people with whom one has a less intimate connection, whereas emotional support involves greater exposure of personal vulnerability. Thus, it is only the people who are closest to the parents and who identify with them with whom they would wish to share their feelings and draw encouragement from. Moreover, while grandparents' ability to provide instrumental assistance may be limited by reasons of health or financial means, such constraints do not hinder their capacity to offer emotional support and afford the parents the sense that they have someone with whom they can share their experiences. This was borne out in a study by Baranowski and Schilmoeller (1999), which showed that mothers of children with disabilities saw the most significant help they received from the grandparents in their "being," rather than "doing,". This attitude was expressed in their study by statements such as: "Always been there for us" (p. 440); "My 'Rock of Gibraltar'" (p. 440); "Always there no matter what" (p. 440); "[My mother] has always loved him unconditionally and treated him with equal affection" (p. 439); and "Always been there for my son" (p. 440).

A study conducted among Israeli mothers of children with a disability (Florian and Findler 2001) found that the instrumental and emotional support received from the grandparents was linked to the former's emotional and marital adjustment. The lack of such support was often associated with poorer adaptation:

I remember that since she was born it was very, very difficult in this aspect, they were simply not there, it was more of calling to ask how was everything, when they came over it was 'hi and bye', but they were not really a part of the experience, which was horrid, just

> *horrid, to walk around with a baby in the hospital, so really, the whole beginning was very, very, very difficult, very lonely, I really do remember the horrible loneliness.* (Mother of a child with a disability)

Similarly, an investigation of American mothers of children with intellectual disability (Heller et al. 2000) revealed a link between a higher level of emotional support from grandparents and a lower level of depression.

Evidently, there is a greater need for instrumental support during the initial period of adjustment, particularly in the case of a severe disability. Over time, when the situation stabilizes and the family has settled into a routine, emotional support becomes more significant. Moreover, as the children grow older, their care requires greater physical effort, which may be difficult for grandparents. However, they can still continue to provide emotional support. These possible explanations gain support from a study that examined the reports of mothers of children with intellectual disability regarding emotional and instrumental assistance from the grandparents at three points in time: childhood, adolescence, and adulthood (Heller et al. 2000). According to the mothers, the grandparents provided the most instrumental support when the children were the youngest.

Cultural perceptions of the grandparents' role may also help to explain differences in the nature of the support they offer. Thus, for example, a study of grandmothers of children with physical disabilities conducted in Panama (Gardner et al. 2004) indicated expressed expectations of instrumental support (economic and medical support), while an Indian study of parents of children with intellectual disability who live with the grandparents revealed that their support reduced the parents' level of both emotional and instrumental stress in regard to their child's care (Upadhyaya and Havalappanavar 2008). While this finding is similar to the results of studies conducted elsewhere, the unique cultural features of Indian society mean that certain types of instrumental support are not possible. For instance, the level of financial stress was not dependent on the degree of grandparents' support since in most cases it is the grandparents who are financially dependent on their children. It is interesting to note that all the parents in this study reported positive support from their own parents, with none indicating that the grandparents were an additional source of stress, as seen in studies in other societies. Here, too, cultural considerations may have influenced parental reports.

4.4 Gender Differences in Utilizing Grandparents' Support

Most investigations of the perceptions of grandparents' support among parents of children with disabilities rely solely on maternal reports. The minority that relates to both parents, views them as a single unit, without distinguishing between mothers and fathers. Only a very few studies have examined the individual perceptions of the two parents. Such an approach is of value, as it recognizes the existence of gender differences in utilizing sources of social support (Trute et al. 2008).

Findings indicate that each of the parents responds in a unique way to grandparental support. Trute (2003) found that the attitude of each parent to the involvement of his or her own mother (but not the mother-in-law) was the strongest predictor of the parent's emotional well-being and stress. Mothers reported lower stress and higher well-being when they received emotional support from their mothers. Fathers' relationships with their mothers was a central factor in their perception of their family life and was associated with fewer symptoms of depression and lower levels of parental stress. A study conducted among 61 couples with a child with developmental disabilities (Sandler et al. 1995) reported similar findings for the fathers, indicating a link between paternal grandparents' support and the emotional adaptation of the father.

When grandparents support their sons or daughters, the latter feel stronger and may consequently have a more positive attitude toward themselves, their family situation, and their partners. Furthermore, the amount of support may increase in the wake of assistance or lack of it from the other set of grandparents, which might create a sense of imbalance. This, in turn, could intensify the feelings of the parent whose own parents are especially helpful or the one whose parents refrain from offering support.

While the studies cited above (Trute 2003; Trute et al. 2008; Sandler et al. 1995) indicate the source of support that contributes most to each of the parents, they do not help in understanding gender differences in the way they are utilized. One study conducted among 34 mothers and 27 fathers of children with Down's syndrome examined the link between support from and conflict with the grandparents on the one hand, and the stress level of each of the parents on the other (Hastings et al. 2002). Both support and conflict were found to predict mother's level of stress, with stress lower among mothers reporting instrumental and emotional support from the grandparents, and higher among those reporting conflicts with the older generation. No significant correlations were found between these variables and father's level of stress. In a longitudinal study (Trute et al. 2008), the associations between maternal and paternal grandmother's support and the coping abilities and stress of each of the parents of children with developmental and intellectual disabilities were examined at two points in time. The first measurement was made on the parents' initial arrival at a diagnostic and treatment center (within six months of registration; all the children were under the age of twelve), and the second, one year later. The findings indicated a link between grandmothers' support and the parental stress of the mother over time, but not of the father.

There are several possible explanations for these gender differences. First, the mother generally bears the greater burden of care for the child, especially in the case of a child with disability. It is therefore reasonable to assume that the mother would be more affected by the grandparents' support, or lack of it, than the father would. Secondly, the literature indicates differences in the utilization of sources of social support. Men and women differ in the nature of their involvement in relationships and in the manner in which they avail themselves of sources of assistance when dealing with stress. While women tend to look to friends and family members for help, men are more likely to focus on a single individual with whom they are in an intimate relationship, most often their partner (Cutrona 1996). Indeed, Trute et al. (2008) found that lower parental stress among fathers was associated with lower parental stress among mothers. Thus, men appear to be particularly sensitive to the parental stress experienced by their wives, and may consequently find it difficult to serve as a source of emotional support for them. However, when the mother receives emotional support from the grandmothers and therefore experiences less parental stress, the father's parental stress is also reduced.

4.5 The Complex Nature of Grandparental Support

Despite the potential value of support from the grandparents in enhancing the well-being and adaptation of parents of a child with a disability, the involvement of their own parents in their lives may sometimes be difficult and constitute a further burden. Parents often welcomed the support and care offered by the grandparents, but they were also frustrated in their desires to perform competently in roles they had assumed for themselves (Nybo et al. 1998). In a study asking parents in these families if the grandparents added to existing problems, 24 % of them responded positively (Hornby and Ashworth 1994). Similarly, when parents of children with epilepsy were asked who provided the minimal support, over 78 % indicated that one of the grandparents provided the least assistance and formed a source of stress and disappointment (Romeis 1980). Thus, when parents' expectations from the grandparents to fulfill a supportive role remain unmet, there is often times a growing sense of estrangement and despair as the following quotes illustrate.

> *My father is not a grandfather, and he will never be a grandfather, he doesn't know what it means to be a grandfather. Of course, when the grandchildren come grandpa gives candies, and grandpa hugs and kisses, but that is it, it ends there. I mean, I wish my children had a grandfather and not only a grandmother.*

> *...My family was disappointing ... I've already given up anger, the anger dissipated, as simple as that, I somehow accept it as it is and that is it.*

> *They never fully understand it, for example, we were in the hospital on Thursday, she was hospitalized with anesthesia, so they were hysterical, calling every half an hour... my mother in law was 'on duty' she took the little one, returned her home, took her to another activity returned her home, like, she is doing and doing, and my family is busy talking my head off, everything is such a drama for them, so as far as I'm concerned, I ask for their help as little as possible, I realized it over the years that I ask as little as possible, and whatever I need I manage with the caregiver and the help of my mother-in-law.*

One of the triggers for tension and anger in families of children with disabilities is the gap between the parents' and the grandparents' perceptions of the child's condition and future. Conflicts may be sharpest when the parents feel that the grandparents are in denial, implying that they do not accept the child for who he or she is and are blind to their special needs, as well as those of the parents (Sandler 1998; Seligman 1991).

> *Perhaps somehow, I think, I did say it to him, in this prickly way, to hurt them, a little bit, like, yes, yes, you have to understand, there is something very, very, big going on over here. I have to tell you, that even today in my conversations with my sisters, with my parents, I'm trying to show them the other side that it seems so trivial to me that my family will be the first to understand, to know and internalize things, but sometimes they don't get it.* (Mother of a child with a disability)

Naturally, parents are likely to experience stress when grandparents' display hostility, confusion, aversion, fear or shame. However, stress may also ensue from remarks that reflect a lack of understanding of the child's disability or doubt as to the need for special treatment, or when grandparents adopt an attitude of unwarranted optimism that denies the reality of the child's condition (Seligman 1991).

Moreover, a study by Gabel and Kotsch (1981) showed that the birth of a child with a disability often forces the parents to support and comfort the grandparents and contend with their disappointment and fears at a time when they themselves are sorely in need of emotional support and encouragement. In such situations, parents may feel a great deal of anger and resentment for having to devote their energy to dealing with their parents' reactions rather than being free to care for the child and cope with their own difficulties.

> *My wife's mother has supported us all along. My wife's father didn't understand us at all, he was really shocked when he first arrived at the special day care, it seemed very odd to him that that was our choice, yet he trusted us because of our knowledge. He said he thought that we probably knew better. Later we also told my father and he responded the same as the other grandfather – 'I don't understand what you want from the child'. How many times can you listen to 'he's perfectly fine, what's the problem?' ...I recall a few times when my wife snapped at her father: "that's how it is, there is a problem, accept it, or at least stop telling us there isn't any". It feels like they need this perfect picture. We needed them in a different way... it is very upsetting that you turn to your father and share with him – "the child undergoes treatments" – and he answers: "everything is alright, you're just being anxious".* (Father of a child with a disability)

Another aspect of the family that may represent an emotional burden for the parents of a child with a disability emerges from a study by Green (2001). The results indicate that when grandparents are incapable of providing active support due to age or other constraints, the parents may be torn between the needs of the child and those of the grandparents, and feel compelled to prove to other family members that they can meet both demands despite the hardship.

Differences in the perception of assistance also add to the complexity of the issue of grandparents' support. Thus, for example, a study comparing the mothers and grandmothers of children on the autism spectrum found discrepancies between the way the two generations perceived the grandmother's role and willingness to help: the grandmothers' perception of their relationship with the grandchild and the part they played in his or her upbringing was more positive than that of their daughters (Sullivan et al. 2012). The authors concluded that mothers are not always aware of the degree to which grandmothers believe they are functioning effectively. Since relationships draw their strength from mutual giving and receiving that fuel one another, differences in the perception of support can be expected to affect both the parents and the grandparents.

> *On the one hand, it's like they are totally there, and they are a supportive, present and conscious family. It's like if you interview them, you'll see the most aware, connected, eloquent and understanding people, not burying their heads in the sand, clearly seeing the disability, trusting the girl and being proud of her, loving her very much, not hiding, talking about it, there's no sense of shame, very open minded. On the other hand, it's like they're living in la-la land... I keep telling my parents take the big one, she's so lonely, take her to a cafe in the afternoon... and with them it's like I'm begging all the time.* (Mother of a child with a disability)

The studies cited above (Green 2001; Sullivan et al. 2012) depict an intricate picture, which makes it clear that grandparents of a child with a disability cannot readily be classified as either a source of support or stress. Furthermore, their assistance cannot be taken for granted. In contrast to other members of the parents' social network (neighbors, friends, etc.), there is a close bond with the grandparents and the relationship between them is emotionally charged. This makes it difficult for parents to adopt a neutral attitude toward them or simply to ignore them when they are not helpful.

By virtue of the family ties, parents in general, and mothers in particular, have expectations of support from their own parents and from their in-laws. If these expectations are not met, the resulting sense of disappointment and frustration is likely to become a source of stress that adversely affects their emotional well-being

> *In her first years, we were preoccupied with her, her, her, her, the preoccupation with her was some sort of a race, and I remember a lot of anger towards my parents, a lot of anger, even when the little one was born, I used to tell my parents, come over, just come and sit here, you don't have to work, you don't have to fold laundry, you don't have to clean up, you don't have to do anything, just come over, enjoy your granddaughters.* (Mother of a child with a disability)

4.6 Factors Predicting Grandparents' Support

Numerous studies have sought to identify the factors that lead to grandparental support, or lack of it, in families of children with disabilities. Investigations have focused, in particular, on the question of whether the presence of such a child in a family affects the level of assistance provided.

A study comparing the support received by mothers of children with spina bifida with those whose children had no disability found that the disability per se was not a factor in the level or type of support provided by the grandparents (Pit-Ten Cate et al. 2007). In a qualitative study of twelve New Zealand families of children with disabilities, both parents and grandparents were questioned regarding mutual relations and support (Mirfin-Veitch et al. 1996; Mirfin-Veitch et al. 1997). In most of the families interviewed, the grandparents provided emotional and instrumental support and expressed a strong sense of belonging and concern for the child's nuclear family in general, and the grandchild in particular. Only a small number of parents reported that the grandparents were distant and uninvolved, and indicated their disappointment with this lack of support. According to the authors, the difference between the two groups was not related to the presence or severity of the disability, but to the history of family relations before the child was born. The birth of a child with a disability accentuated the existing relationship, so that previous intimacy and open communications between the parents and grandparents gave rise to empathy and more emotional and instrumental support after the child's birth. On the other hand, where the relationship had been distant and cold, the birth of the child led to even greater distance, lack of assistance, and estrangement. Similar findings emerged from a study of 105 mothers of children with cerebral palsy, which showed a strong association between grandparents' support and their closeness to their children before the birth of the grandchild (Baranowski and Schilmoeller 1999).

A particularly interesting finding was produced by a study that sought to investigate the perceptions of mothers of children with disabilities toward their parents and their spouses' parents regarding the support they provide. The participants were asked to respond with reference to two time points: "before" (the disability became apparent) and "now" (Seligman et al. 1997). Mothers' reports revealed that although they sensed no change in the level of support they received from their own parents, there was a significant increase in support from their in-laws once the disability became known (Seligman et al. 1997). The birth of a child with a disability may very well have sparked the in-laws' awareness of the importance of their assistance, which was then manifested in a greater willingness to help out. It is also possible that the mother took support from her parents for granted, whereas she did not have a similar expectation from her in-laws. Thus, she might have been more conscious of any support they did provide.

> *My son's grandmother from my husband's side is an amazing grandmother, nothing compares to her, she helps, always is available, she loves my son as if he were her son, and she will give him absolutely everything. First of all, he is the first grandson, so that's for her — In my family, my son was maybe the sixteenth, fifteenth, grandson, so it's like a little different... I think it's different with the first grandson in terms of acceptance, my husband's mother does not move away from him, she spent a lot of time with us in the hospitals, in many places, and she also lives nearby, so that's very helpful. My mother, after having raised so many children and grandchildren, although she really loves my son, she's not available, she works a lot, she's too busy to see him, we see her once a week, and she loves him a lot, but it's different, no doubt it's different. Usually it's the other way around, it's my mother who is supposed to help us more than his mother, usually that is the case but for us it's different, it's because we live closer to her [mother in law], and, also because she is younger in spirit, more flexible, it's easier with her... To be honest, it's also easier for me to talk to my husband's mother, because if I talk to my mother she takes things very, very hard. She becomes very sad in no time and I do not want to cause it, it's unfair... My husband's mother is there for us much more than my mother. Again, perhaps if we had lived closer it would be different, but I doubt it, my mother in law is amazing, and that's what I love about her, so much patience she has, it's incredible, it's great.* (Mother of a child with a disability)

While most studies above (Baranowski and Schilmoeller 1999; Mirfin-Veitch et al. 1996; Mirfin-Veitch et al. 1997; Pit-ten Cate et al. 2007) indicated that, on the whole, the presence of a child with a disability did not have a critical effect on the support received from the grandparents, a qualitative study conducted in Sweden among thirteen parents of children with disabilities found that the child's condition strengthened the family unit and led to increased grandparental support (Lindblad et al. 2007). The parents reported closer ties with their parents, and stated that the grandparents' acceptance of the child's condition helped all sides to view their new reality as part of the current family story, and enhanced their sense of togetherness. It is possible, however, that the families in this study enjoyed positive and mutually supportive relationships prior to the child's birth and that the greater degree of support provided after the birth was the outcome of a close family bonding. In other words, it was not the child's disability itself that created a support system inside the family, but rather the family relations prior to the birth.

This explanation would be consistent with the findings presented above regarding the association between grandparents' support and the pre-existing family relationship (Baranowski and Schilmoeller 1999; Mirfin-Veitch et al. 1996, 1997; Pit-ten Cate et al. 2007).

According to Fischer (1983), geographical closeness and maternal kinship tend to be indicators of a strong grandchild-grandmother relationship. Pit-Ten Cate et al. (2007) found that the geographical distance was associated with grandmother's degree of support: residential proximity to paternal grandparents was related to perceived support from both maternal and paternal grandparents. In other words, grandparents who live close to a grandchild with a disability appear more likely to make themselves accessible and open to learning skills and performing activities that provide direct support for their grandchild's family system (Gardner et al. 1994). It is worth emphasizing that although physical distance often prevented instrumental support (Gardner et al. 1994), it did not necessarily prevent grandparents from providing emotional one.

> *I believe that if I need my Mom's help she will definitely say yes, but it must be on her terms, that I will have to bring him to her ...My Mom knows she doesn't help me, she tells me: "I wish I could do more, but you're far away from me".* (Mother of a child with a disability)

4.7 The Differential Contribution of Each of the Grandparents

Grandparents can be a stable and significant component of any family's support system, and their contribution to the family of a child with a disability may be invaluable. Indeed, when mothers of children with disabilities are asked to evaluate the support of the significant individuals in their social support network, all the grandparents feature high on the scale of importance (Hornby and Ashworth 1994;

Sharpley et al. 1997). However, the four grandparents do not present a homogenous picture in terms of the support they provide to the family, and should not be seen as a single unit.

Mothers who were asked to rank the degree of support they received from the different grandparents revealed that although both pairs of grandparents helped, the maternal grandmother was most often ranked the highest (Seligman et al. 1997; Shaw 2005; Trute 2003; Trute et al. 2008), followed in order by the maternal grandfather, the paternal grandmother, and finally, the paternal grandfather. Similar findings emerged from an Israeli study in which mothers of children with disabilities were asked to rank the importance of twelve significant support figures (Findler 2000). The maternal grandmother was placed first, followed by the maternal grandfather (5), the paternal grandmother (8), and the paternal grandfather (11). In a study conducted in Britain, mothers also reported receiving more support from their own parents than from their in-laws (Pit-ten Cate et al. 2007). The greater support offered to families of children with disabilities by the maternal grandparents, as compared to the paternal grandparents, is expressed mainly in more positive attitudes and greater empathy, but is also reflected in the extent and frequency of support (Baranowski and Schilmoeller 1999; Bruns and Foerster 2011; Hornby and Ashworth 1994).

> *Mostly the help comes from my wife's parents, my wife's parents were our source of advice [after the diagnosis] and the reactions were different: the father was against putting the kid in a special day care. The grandmother immediately joined a grandparents' group, she went ahead with it straight away realizing that that's what we needed, this kind of support, so she was present at most of the consultations, asking questions or just talking. Until today she's the most involved grandmother in my son's treatment.* (Father of a child with a disability)

Thus, in view of the hardship typically experienced by families of children with disabilities, the maternal grandparents appear to play a major and highly significant role in the life of the mother, who generally endures the most of the child's care. As described in chapter three, the literature relates to the strong bond between the mother and her parents from the perspective of the grandparents as well. The preference for the daughter's family over that of the son runs like a thread throughout both empirical research and clinical descriptions (Findler 2000; Vadasy et al. 1986). An Israeli study found that mothers of children with typical development and mothers of children with a physical disability indicated more support from both maternal grandparents than from either paternal grandparent (Findler 2000). Similarly, in an examination of the support and involvement of grandparents in families of Deafblind children, mothers ranked the maternal grandmother highest, followed by the maternal grandfather followed by paternal grandmother and last in the list was the paternal grandfather (Shaw 2005). In another study, mothers of children with disability defined their own mother as their primary source of emotional support, that is, the person they could speak to and who would listen and offer encouragement (Baranowski and Schilmoeller 1999).

The special place occupied by the maternal grandparents in general, and the maternal grandmother in particular, can be accounted for in various ways.

A common approach holds that the middle generation is largely responsible for the tri-generational connection, and that the mother is the most active in relations with the extended family. By nature, it is easier for her to turn first to her family of origin, and especially her mother (Bowen 1978). As described in chapter three, the explanation for the close bond between a daughter and her mother derives from psychoanalytic theory, which holds that the basic affinity for the mother generally remains intact and becomes an important and productive part of a woman's world throughout her life. When she herself becomes a mother, her respect for and closeness to her own mother grow stronger, and her dependence on her takes on a more mature nature (Fischer 1983).

A study conducted in the US among parents and grandparents of children with autism (Glasberg and Harris 1997) lends support to Bowen's (1978) theory. It showed, on the one hand, that there were differences in perceptions between the generations with regard to the child's condition. On the other hand, however, it was indicated that the maternal grandparents' standpoints were generally closer to those of the parents' than the paternal grandparents' views. The discrepancy between the perceptions of the parents and the paternal grandparents came to the fore in the latter's overly optimistic view of the child's abilities. The authors suggested that this gap stems from the different degrees of involvement of either set of grandparents.

One study, however, presents the mother-in-law in a more positive light, reporting that grandmothers on both sides provide more support than grandfathers do - especially emotional support. Paternal grandmother's emotional support, in addition to that of the maternal grandmother, was found to be a major factor in reducing the level of stress among the mothers of children with disabilities in the study (Trute et al. 2008).

As suggested above, it may be that due to her ongoing distress, the mother of a child with a disability is more in need of her parents and feels more comfortable accepting their assistance. On the other hand, routine help with a child with typical development is welcomed more readily from both grandmothers, who may themselves feel more at ease with the child and capable of caring for them.

In view of the literature, it is evident that grandparents may perform a significant role in families of children with disabilities, either as a major source of support or as a potential source of stress. Whatever the role is, it has a strong impact on the nuclear family. Research points at the complex emotional experience of both providing and receiving support on the part of the grandparents and parents respectively. Furthermore, research indicates that the four grandparents do not constitute one coherent unit and therefore, the nature and extent of such support, if any, vary from one grandparent to another.

The potential value of the contribution of grandmothers and grandfathers to the support system of families of children with disabilities cannot be underestimated. When professionals formulate intervention programs with parents, it is vital that they keep in mind the importance of the grandparents' role. It is advisable that professionals also encourage parents to allow and develop effective communication channels with the grandparents in order to enable and nurture this meaningful support resource for the benefit of the intergenerational relationships in the family.

References

Baranowski, M. D., & Schilmoeller, G. L. (1999). Grandparents in the lives of grandchildren with disabilities: Mothers' perceptions. *Education & Treatment of Children, 22*, 427–446.

Barnett, W. S., & Boyce, G. C. (1995). Effects of children with Down syndrome on parents' activities. *American Journal on mental Retardation, 100*, 115–127.

Bowen, M. (1978). *Family therapy in clinical practice*. Lanham, MD: Jason Aronson.

Bruns, D., & Foerster, K. (2011). "We've been through it all together": Supports for parents with children with rare trisomy conditions. *Journal of Intellectual Disability Research, 55*, 361–369.

Case-Smith, J. (2012). Parenting a child with a chronic medical condition. In I. Marini & M. A. Stebnicki (Eds.), *The psychological and social impact of illness and disability* (pp. 219–231). New York, NY: Springer Publishing.

Crnic, K. A., Friedrich, W. N., & Greenberg, M. T. (1983). Adaptation of families with mentally retarded children: A model of stress, coping, and family ecology. *American Journal of Mental Deficiency, 88*, 125–138.

Cutrona, C. E. (1996). Social support as a determinant of marital quality: The interplay of negative and supportive behaviors. In G. R. Pierce, B. R. Sarason, & I. G. Sarason (Eds.), *Handbook of social support and the family: Plenum series on stress and coping* (pp. 173–194). New York, NY: Plenum Press.

Findler, L. (2000). The role of grandparents in the social support system of mothers of children with a physical disability. *Families in Society, 81*, 370–381.

Findler, L. (2014). The experience of stress and personal growth among grandparents of children with and without intellectual disability. *Intellectual and Developmental Disabilities, 52*, 32–48.

Finzi-Dottan, R., Triwitz, Y. S., & Golubchik, P. (2011). Predictors of stress-related growth in parents of children with ADHD. *Research in Developmental Disabilities, 32*, 510–519.

Fischer, L. R. (1983). Transition to grandmotherhood. *The International Journal of Aging & Human Development, 16*, 67–78.

Florian, V., & Findler, L. (2001). Mental health and marital adaptation among mothers of children with cerebral palsy. *American Journal of Orthopsychiatry, 71*, 358–367.

Friedrich, W. N., & Friedrich, W. L. (1981). Psychosocial assets of parents of handicapped and non-handicapped children. *American Journal of Mental Deficiency, 85*, 551–553.

Gabel, H., & Kotsch, L. S. (1981). Extended families and young handicapped children. *Topics in Early Childhood Special Education, 1*, 29–35.

Gardner, J. E., Scherman, A., Efthimiadis, M. S., & Shultz, S. K. (2004). Panamanian grandmothers' family relationships and adjustment to having a grandchild with a disability. *The International Journal of Aging & Human Development, 59*, 305–320.

Gardner, J. E., Scherman, A., Mobley, D., Brown, P., & Schutter, M. (1994). Grandparents' beliefs regarding their role and relationship with special needs grandchildren. *Education & Treatment of Children, 17*, 185–196.

Glasberg, B. A., & Harris, S. L. (1997). Grandparents and parents assess the development of their child with autism. *Child & Family Behavior Therapy, 19*, 17–27.

Glidden, L. M., & Schoolcraft, S. A. (2003). Depression: Its trajectory and correlates in mothers rearing children with intellectual disability. *Journal of Intellectual Disability Research, 47*, 250–263.

Green, S. E. (2001). Grandma's hands: Parental perceptions of the importance of grandparents as secondary caregivers in families of children with disabilities. *The International Journal of Aging & Human Development, 53*, 11–33.

Hastings, R. P., Thomas, H., & Delwiche, N. (2002). Grandparent support for families of children with Down's syndrome. *Journal of Applied Research in Intellectual Disabilities, 15*, 97–104.

Heller, T., Hsieh, K., & Rowitz, L. (2000). Grandparents as supports to mothers of persons with intellectual disability. *Journal of Gerontological Social Work, 33*, 23–34.

Hillman, J. (2007). Grandparents of children with autism: A review with recommendations for education, practice, and policy. *Educational Gerontology, 33*, 513–527.

Hornby, G., & Ashworth, T. (1994). Grandparents' support for families who have children with disabilities. *Journal of Child and Family Studies, 3*, 403–412.

Katz, S., & Kessel, L. (2002). Grandparents of children with developmental disabilities: Perceptions, beliefs, and involvement in their care. *Issues in Comprehensive Pediatric Nursing, 25*, 113–128.

Kornhaber, A. (1986). Grandparenting: Normal and pathological: A preliminary communication from The Grandparent Study. *Journal of Geriatric Psychiatry, 19*, 19–37.

Larson, E. (2010). Psychological well-being and meaning-making when caregiving for children with disabilities: Growth through difficult times or sinking inward. *OTJR: Occupation Participation and Health, 30*, 78–86.

Lee, M., & Gardner, J. E. (2010). Grandparents' involvement and support in families with children with disabilities. *Educational Gerontology, 36*, 467–499.

Lindblad, B. M., Holritz-Rasmussen, B., & Sandman, P. O. (2007). A life enriching togetherness—Meanings of informal support when being a parent of a child with disability. *Scandinavian Journal of Caring Sciences, 21*, 238–246.

Manor-Binyamini, I. (2014). Positive aspects of the coping of mothers of adolescent children with developmental disability in the Bedouin community in Israel. *Research in Developmental Disabilities, 35*, 1272–1280.

Mirfin-Veitch, B., Bray, A., & Watson, M. (1996). "They really do care": Grandparents as informal support sources for families of children with disabilities. *New Zealand Journal of Disability Studies, 2*, 136–148.

Mirfin-Veitch, B., Bray, A., & Watson, M. (1997). "We're just that sort of family": Intergenerational relationships in families including children with disabilities. *Family Relations: Interdisciplinary Journal of Applied Family Studies, 46*, 305–311.

Nybo, W. L., Scherman, A., & Freeman, P. L. (1998). Grandparents' role in family systems with a deaf child: An exploratory study. *American Annals of the Deaf, 143*, 260–267.

Pit-Ten Cate, I. M., Hastings, R. P., Johnson, H., & Titus, S. (2007). Grandparent support for mothers of children with and without physical disabilities. *Families in Society, 88*, 141–146.

Resch, J. A., Benz, M. R., & Elliott, T. R. (2012). Evaluating a dynamic process model of wellbeing for parents of children with disabilities: A multi-method analysis. *Rehabilitation Psychology, 57*, 61–72.

Romeis, J. C. (1980). The role of grandparents in adjustment to epilepsy. *Social Work in Health Care, 6*, 37–43.

Sandler, A. G. (1998). Grandparents of children with disabilities: A closer look. *Education and Training in Mental Retardation and Developmental Disabilities, 33*, 350–356.

Sandler, A. G., Warren, S. H., & Raver, S. A. (1995). Grandparents as a source of support for parents of children with disabilities: A brief report. *Mental Retardation, 33*, 248–250.

Seligman, M. (1991). Grandparents of disabled grandchildren: Hopes, fears, and adaptation. *Families in Society, 72*, 147–152.

Seligman, M., Goodwin, G., Paschal, K., Applegate, A., & Lehman, L. (1997). Grandparents of children with disabilities: Perceived levels of support. *Education & Training in Mental Retardation & Developmental Disabilities, 32*, 293–303.

Sharpley, C. F., Bitsika, V., & Efremidis, B. (1997). Influence of gender, parental health, and perceived expertise of assistance upon stress, anxiety, and depression among parents of children with autism. *Journal of Intellectual and Developmental Disability, 22*, 19–28.

Shaw, S. L. (2005). Grandparent involvement in the communication development of children who are deafblind. *Educational Gerontology, 31*, 51–71.

Sullivan, A., Winograd, G., Verkuilen, J., & Fish, M. C. (2012). Children on the autism spectrum: Grandmother involvement and family functioning. *Journal of Applied Research in Intellectual Disabilities, 25*, 484–494.

Tak, Y. R., & McCubbin, M. (2002). Family stress, perceived social support and coping following the diagnosis of a child with congenital heart disease. *Journal of Advanced Nursing, 39*, 190–198.

Thomas, J. L. (1990). The grandparent role: A double bind. *The International Journal of Aging & Human Development, 31*, 169–177.

Trute, B. (2003). Grandparents of children with developmental disabilities: Intergenerational support and family well-being. *Families in Society, 84*, 119–126.

Trute, B., Worthington, C., & Hiebert-Murphy, D. (2008). Grandmother support for parents of children with disabilities: Gender differences in parenting stress. *Families systems & health, 26*, 135–146.

Upadhyaya, G. R., & Havalappanavar, N. B. (2008). Grandparental support for parents of mentally retarded children. *Journal of the Indian Academy of Applied Psychology, 34*, 137–141.

Vadasy, P. F. (1987). Grandparents of children with special needs: Supports especially for grandparents. *Children's Health Care, 16*, 21–23.

Vadasy, P. F., Fewell, R. R., & Meyer, D. J. (1986). Grandparents of children with special needs: Insight into their experience and concerns. *Journal of Early Intervention, 10*, 36–44.

Wolfensberger, W., & Menolascino, F. J. (1970). A theoretical framework for the management of parents of the mentally retarded. W. Wolfensberger & F. J. Menolascino, (Eds.), *Psychiatric approaches to mental retardation* (pp. 475–493). New York, NY: Basic Books.

Chapter 5
Twice Special—Grandparents Who Raise Grandchildren with Disabilities

Adi Noy and Liora Findler

Abstract The phenomenon of grandparents, mostly grandmothers, raising a grandchild with a disability has been growing in recent decades. Taking over the parental function, whether temporarily or permanently, entails considerable burdens and has far-reaching implications on both the personal and interpersonal levels. Such grandparents experience physical and emotional challenges, all the more so when dealing with a child with a disability whose needs often require additional resources. In many cases, their status is not legally or formally defined, and they may therefore 'fall between the cracks', leaving them with neither clear legal status nor group affiliation. The chapter describes the characteristics of these grandparents, as well as the particular needs arising from the task of raising a grandchild with a disability, and the costs and benefits of this role. In addition, it discusses the ways in which these grandparents make use of community services and other formal sources of support.

Keywords Grandparenthood · Grandparents of children with a disability · Grandparents raising their grandchildren · Formal social support

In the prevalent discourse, the grandparents' place in the intergenerational family context of grandparents-parents-grandchildren is typically mediated by the parents. Various circumstances, however, may make it impossible for the parents to raise their own children. In such cases, the grandparents may be called upon to fulfill the primary role in the child's life.

Grandparents, who raise their grandchildren, perform all the parental functions, either temporarily or permanently, serving as substitutes for parents who are unable to care for their children. This situation may result from a variety of reasons, including teenage pregnancy, substance abuse, AIDS, child abuse (violence, neglect), imprisonment, abandonment, the parent's physical or cognitive disabilities, or their untimely death (Force et al. 2000; Gallagher et al. 2010).

In recent decades, the phenomenon of grandparents raising their grandchildren has been growing. It is estimated that there are 2.7 million in the US, 200,000 in Great Britain, and 22,500 in Australia (Harnett et al. 2014; Lee and Blitz 2014). Although they can be found in diverse social strata and different ethnic groups, in

L. Findler and O. Taubman – Ben-Ari, *Grandparents of Children with Disabilities*, SpringerBriefs in Well-Being and Quality of Life Research,
DOI 10.1007/978-3-319-45517-4_5

the US they are especially prevalent among African-American and Hispanic minorities (Rubin 2013).

Due to the increase in life expectancy, grandparents have become more actively involved in their grandchildren's lives for a longer period of time, and thus today may be more capable of replacing parents who are unable to raise their children. Moreover, changes in family structure in modern society have given rise to an increasing number of single-parent families. This situation often incurs financial difficulties, with the consequent need to work full-time outside the home. Given the scarcity of appropriate community frameworks for the children, more grandparents have assumed the role of custodians in these families (Force et al. 2000; Gallagher et al. 2010).

While the number of grandparents raising grandchildren, with or without disabilities, has been growing, studies indicate that the features of the role have remained largely unchanged over time. These include the grandparents' characteristics and needs, and the costs and benefits associated with fulfilling this role.

The characteristics of grandparents raising their grandchildren vary widely, perhaps due to the diversity of their cultural origins and socio-demographic traits (Rubin 2013). On the whole, however, it can be said that the majority are women under the age of 65 whose economic condition is poor (Hayslip and Kaminski 2005), and that compared to caregivers in foster homes, they are older and less educated (Harnett et al. 2014). Yet despite the heterogeneity of their personal characteristics, there is considerable similarity among grandparents who raise their grandchildren with regard to their perception of the costs and benefits of their role.

5.1 The Costs and Benefits of Raising Grandchildren

Being the primary caretaker for a grandchild is fundamentally different from the traditional role of grandparents. It entails a heavy workload and substantial investment of time, energy, and money. Performing the parental functions includes responsibility for the grandchild's physical, mental, educational, and social needs. In order to provide for these needs, the grandparents must allocate time and patience, and have to be involved in school programs and after-school activities. This may require them to acquire knowledge of domains that have changed since their own children were young. Taking care of a grandchild may also pose physical challenges, especially if the child is young child or has a disability.

Research shows that many grandparents are seriously conflicted, as they did not anticipate having to raise their grandchild and feel they were trapped into a commitment they could not refuse. In fact, many feel that they had no choice in the matter, since they did not want the child to be raised in foster homes among strangers (Shakya et al. 2012).

As opposed to caregiving in formal foster homes, the task of raising a grandchild often occurs without prior planning (Hayslip and Kaminski 2005). This may explain the high level of stress these grandparents experience, compared to caregivers in foster homes (Harnett et al. 2014). The personal implications on the grandparents' lives are profound, and may include damage to their physical and mental well-being, as well as to their economic situation. Indeed, grandparents who are raising their grandchildren report a higher occurrence of physical and mental illness, including high blood pressure, diabetes, sleeping problems, and depression, than those who are not (Hayslip and Kaminski 2005). It has also been found that since these grandparents feel obligated to put the child's needs first, they tend to neglect their own needs, especially their health. Their commitment to the child also reduces their economic resources, both due to the additional expense of raising the grandchild and the difficulty of working at the same time. Furthermore, the aging process intensifies their concerns about the grandchild's future, particularly after their death (Lee and Blitz 2014).

Raising a grandchild is also seen to place additional pressure on the spousal relationship. Moreover, grandparents who raise their grandchildren express feelings of isolation both from their peers who do not fulfill a similar role, and from parents of young children (Hayslip and Kaminski 2005). In addition, the grandparents' relationship with the grandchild they are raising and their other grandchildren is marked by confusion and conflicting roles. They typically express the desire to be able to play the kind, loving, and indulgent grandparent for the child they were raising as well, and feel a sense of loss at being forced to assume the authoritative role of the parent (Lee and Blitz 2014).

Furthermore, the grandparents are often faced with the additional difficulty of dealing with the absence of their own child from the grandchild's life. When the situation results from the death of the parent, the grandparents must contend with the mourning of their child at the same time as the grandchild is mourning the loss of his parent. Some grandparents find it hard to express their grief and accept support from family members and friends. Alternatively, they may feel that their mourning is not acknowledged by society due to the particular circumstances of their child's absence or death, and may themselves suffer guilt or shame because of these circumstances (Hayslip and Kaminski 2005).

Families where the parent is not completely absent but whose presence is erratic may experience another stress factor: the parent's relationship with the child on the one hand, and with the grandparents on the other. Relations with the grandparents may often be strained and characterized by guilt, anger, and sorrow. Indeed, studies show that the better the grandparents' relationship with the parent, the less likely they are to experience a sense of burden (Hayslip and Kaminski 2005). Grandparents report feeling guilt and shame over their child's failure as a parent and the severe impact of their unstable conduct on the grandchild. They are frequently forced to mediate between the parent and the child, and suffer the negative consequences of the parent's irregular involvement. The parent tends to show up sporadically and unannounced, behavior that may result from engaging in casual romantic relationships or drug abuse (Shakya et al. 2012).

A further stress factor indicated by grandparents is the generation gap. They are highly sensitive to the age gap between themselves and their grandchildren, as well as to differences in the accepted parenting style since they were raising their own children. Most of them feel that the changes that have occurred over time are negative and conflict with their values, and are concerned about the influence on their grandchild's upbringing (Shakya et al. 2012).

As raising grandchildren is a complex experience that requires considerable coping skills, these grandparents are typically in need of support. Nonetheless, they note a failure to receive sufficient emotional and instrumental support (Harnett et al. 2014). A recurrent finding indicates that these grandparents rarely use community services, and that, in fact, few services are available to them (Harnett et al. 2014; Janicki et al. 2000; Shakya et al. 2012; Yancura 2013). A study conducted in the US, for example, showed that one third of grandparents raising their grandchildren had insufficient information about their rights and did not receive an adequate response to the grandchildren's needs in regard to tutoring and extra-curricular activities (Yancura 2013). The problem is therefore two-pronged: on the one hand, grandparents do not, of their own volition, request assistance; and on the other hand, the services available to them are limited and not compatible with their needs.

One explanation for the grandparents' reluctance to make use of community services is their apprehension that welfare authorities might intervene in their life, and specifically in their decision to take over responsibility for their grandchild (Harnett et al. 2014). Grandparents often express the concern that they might be deemed unfit to raise their grandchildren, and that the children might be removed from their care and transferred to foster homes. Many also report that interacting with the authorities is overly complicated for them. Obstacles related to accessibility, such as scheduling meetings with the proper officials, make it more difficult to use the services that are available. Naturally, when the grandparents' formal legal status is not clearly defined, the receipt of these services becomes even more complicated (Janicki et al. 2000; Shakya et al. 2012).

Alongside the high costs of raising grandchildren, the role may be extremely rewarding as it involves a close, satisfying, and enriching relationship with the child. Most grandparents who raise their grandchildren report that if they had to do it all over again, they would make the same choice to raise their grandchildren, since it provides them with a sense of purpose and the satisfaction of knowing they are preserving their family's integrity (Hayslip and Kaminski 2005). The majority regard the experience as a second chance to fulfill the parental role, this time with greater understanding which enables them to avoid some of the pitfalls of their own earlier parenting, and as an opportunity to heal past "wounds" when raising their own children (Lee and Blitz 2014). Grandmothers perceive themselves as wiser, calmer, and more actively involved in their children's upbringing than they were with own children (Dolbin-MacNab 2006).

The grandchildren may also gain from being raised by their grandparents. When the nuclear family falls apart, the grandparents represent security, and serve as a safety net and a source of love and warmth for the children (Hayslip and Kaminski 2005). Grandchildren raised by their grandparents adapt better to their new family circumstances and behave more positively than children in foster homes (Harnett et al. 2014). However, compared to children brought up by their parents, they are often raised in poverty, lack medical care, and have problems with school registration since their grandparents' legal status is unclear (Hayslip et al. 2014).

5.2 Raising a Grandchild with a Disability

The circumstances which lead grandparents to raise their grandchildren are naturally more stressful and challenging in the case of a child with a disability, and even more so when the child's disability is the outcome of the parents' maladaptive behavior (Gallagher et al. 2010). Substance abuse, along with the consequent possibility of premature birth, as well as abuse, neglect, malnutrition, and deprivation of stimuli in the infant's early years may all result in intellectual and developmental disabilities (Janicki et al. 2000), including learning disabilities, developmental delays, ADHD, speech or hearing impairment, and neurological problems (Neely-Barnes and Dia 2008).

The characteristics of grandparents raising grandchildren with and without disabilities are similar. Generally, they are grandmothers (over 90 %), belong to minority groups (for example, African-American, Hispanic), are in their late fifties or early sixties, have a high school education, and live in urban areas (Neely-Barnes and Dia 2008). No differences have been found between grandmothers who raise children with and without disabilities in regard to their age, the grandchild's age, education, ethnicity, or family status. There does appear to be a difference, however, in terms of income, as grandmothers raising grandchildren with disabilities tend to have a lower income (Kresak et al. 2014). Often, their socio-economic status renders them unable to afford after-school assistance (Gallagher et al. 2010). The economic burden is especially heavy due both to the added expense of the grandchild's care and the inability to work outside the home (Rubin 2013). Grandparents who raise children with disabilities also report poorer health than those raising children without disabilities (Burnette 2000).

While all grandparents who serve as the primary caretakers for their grandchildren have a lot in common, raising a grandchild with a disability poses unique challenges. The similarity stems from the shared demands of caring for a young child and concerns about being perceived as unfit. When the specific difficulties of raising a child with a disability are added to the burden, studies show that grandparents who raise their grandchildren, like parents, often feel overwhelmed (Janicki et al. 2000). Similar to parents who learn that their child has a disability, accepting the reality that the grandchild is not what they hoped and dreamed of is likely to be a lengthy process. Although the first encounter with the grandchild is often accompanied by a sense of concern, fear, sadness, and helplessness, in time most grandparents adjust and feelings of acceptance, hopefulness, and other positive emotions emerge (Schilmoeller and Baranowski 1998).

Grandparents who raise their grandchildren are naturally concerned about the child's future, when they will no longer be able to care for them. It goes without saying that these concerns are intensified when the grandchild's disability imposes greater dependence. Worried about the grandchild's ability to manage on their own, the grandparents are acutely aware of their advancing age and of the fact that the child will need other caregivers in the future (Janicki et al. 2000).

Moreover, fulfilling the parental role for a grandchild with a disability exacts considerable personal costs. Due to their profound commitment to the child, grandparents' resources are directed to the youngster's needs rather than to their own. They rarely have free time for themselves or to meet with family and friends, and often find themselves outside the social circle of their peers as they are unable to participate in social events, to travel, etc. Furthermore, they not only neglect their health, but actively try to hide health problems lest they be deemed unfit to raise their grandchildren (Janicki et al. 2000).

The heavy burden of raising a grandchild with a disability (Conway et al. 2010) frequently manifests in depression (Musil et al. 2009). Indeed, while it has been found that grandparents who raised their grandchildren with and without disabilities experience higher levels of depression than their peers (Force et al. 2000), African-American grandmothers raising grandchildren with disabilities report even greater depression than those raising grandchildren without disabilities (Kolomer et al. 2002). Grandmothers who raise children with disabilities also display less satisfaction with all dimensions of their family's quality of life, save for the parental role (Kresak et al. 2014).

Similar to the picture that emerges for parents, the level of distress among grandmothers who raise grandchildren is predicted by behavior problems exhibited by the grandchildren (Kelley et al. 2011), with more behavioral problems linked to a heavier emotional burden (Conway et al. 2011) and higher levels of distress (Kelley et al. 2013) among the grandmothers. Moreover, the grandchildren's mental and behavioral difficulties have been found to predict both the grandparent's personal distress and the distress associated with the parental role they fulfill (Hayslip et al. 2014). This is further indication of the heavier toll taken on grandparents raising a child with a disability.

5.3 The Unique Needs of Grandparents Who Raise Grandchildren with Disabilities

Raising a grandchild with a cognitive or physical disability entails the need to provide the child with the appropriate care. Many such children also exhibit behavioral problems in school, and a large percentage of grandparents admit being concerned about this behavior and having difficulty dealing with it. They report being unable to leave the child alone or in the care of another person, experiencing sleep problems, and facing physical challenges, such as lifting the child or carrying them up and down stairs (Janicki et al. 2000).

Grandmothers raising grandchildren with disabilities refer to the need for specific information or guidance for dealing with issues such as behavioral problems or language difficulties related to the grandchild's disability. They indicate that when they do receive this information, it helps them to respond to the grandchild's needs. In particular, the grandmothers express a desire for information regarding the grandchild's experience in his or her special education school, since many of them were not actively involved in the child's school program prior to assuming parental responsibilities. In addition, those who are also raising the siblings of a grandchild with a disability speak of a need for instructive information regarding the relationship between the children (Gallagher et al. 2010).

Other needs mentioned by grandparents of children with disabilities are linked to the formal and informal support systems. They refer to the need for support from formal support systems to assist in advancing the grandchild's development, as well as the desire for an informal support system that connects them with other grandparents facing similar challenges and may provide emotional and instrumental support (Gallagher et al. 2010).

Although the extra burden of raising a grandchild with a disability incurs an enhanced need for support, it appears that such grandparents enjoy little assistance and guidance. In fact, a comparative study found that grandparents raising a child with a disability used community services to a lesser degree than those raising a child without a disability. Only 10 % of grandmothers who raised children with disabilities were in contact with community services (Force et al. 2000). Furthermore, they received significantly less informal support than grandparents raising children without disabilities. The reason for the discrepancy may lie in the difficulty of family members and friends to deal with the disability and consequently to be supportive (Kresak et al. 2014).

Little or no support has serious implications for grandparents in general, and those raising a child with a disability in particular. Research indicates that greater burden along with insufficient support, both of which characterize grandparents raising a child with a disability, are associated with a higher level of depression (Musil et al. 2009). Conversely, greater assistance with the child has been shown to correlate negatively with depression, stress, and anxiety, and positively with higher life satisfaction (Doley et al. 2015) and a higher level of satisfaction with family life (Kresak et al. 2014).

To conclude, the phenomenon of grandparents, mostly grandmothers, raising children with disabilities has been growing in recent decades. Often, their (grand) parental status is not defined legally or formally, leaving them with neither clear legal status nor group affiliation. This population has also received little theoretical, research, and clinical attention. Nevertheless, the challenges facing them are daunting, and their custodial responsibilities have far-reaching implications on both the personal and interpersonal levels. The physical and emotional difficulties of raising a child at an advanced age are even greater when the child has a disability, and therefore more resources of all sorts are required to meet their needs. Given these circumstances, the grandparents need the support of both formal and informal support systems. Yet their use of such services is infrequent, creating a paradoxical situation in which the people with an enhanced need for support receive far less than other populations. Clearly, professionals must step in here to provide an appropriate response for these grandparents that will assist them in performing their highly challenging role.

References

Burnette, D. (2000). Latino grandparents rearing grandchildren with special needs: Effects on depressive symptomatology. In P. McCallion & M. Janicki (Eds.), *Grandparents as carers of children with disabilities: Facing the challenges* (pp. 1–16). Binghamton, NY: The Haworth Press Inc.

Conway, F., Jones, S., & Speakes-Lewis, A. (2011). Emotional strain in caregiving among African American grandmothers raising their grandchildren. *Journal of Women & Aging, 23*, 113–128.

Conway, P., Boeckel, J., Shuster, L., & Wages, J. (2010). Grandparent caregivers' use of resources and services, level of burden, and factors that mediate their relationships. *Journal of Intergenerational Relationships, 8*, 128–144.

Dolbin-MacNab, M. L. (2006). Just like raising your own? Grandmothers' perceptions of parenting a second time around. *Family Relations: An Interdisciplinary Journal of Applied Family Studies, 55*, 564–575.

Doley, R., Bell, R., Watt, B., & Simpson, H. (2015). Grandparents raising grandchildren: Investigating factors associated with distress among custodial grandparent. *Journal of Family Studies, 21*, 101–119.

Force, L. T., Botsford, A., Pisano, P. A., & Holbert, A. (2000). Grandparents raising children with and without a developmental disability: Preliminary comparisons. *Journal of Gerontological Social Work, 33*, 5–21.

Gallagher, P. A., Kresak, K., & Rhodes, C. A. (2010). Perceived needs of grandmothers of children with disabilities. *Topics in Early Childhood Special Education, 30*, 56–64.

Harnett, P. H., Dawe, S., & Russell, M. (2014). An investigation of the needs of grandparents who are raising grandchildren. *Child and Family Social Work, 19*, 411–420.

Hayslip, B., Blumenthal, H., & Garner, A. (2014). Health and grandparent—grandchild well-being: One-year longitudinal findings for custodial grand families. *Journal of Aging and Health, 26*, 559–582.

Hayslip, B., & Kaminski, P. L. (2005). Grandparents raising their grandchildren: A review of the literature and suggestions for practice. *The Gerontologist, 45*, 262–269.

Janicki, M. P., McCallion, P., Grant-Griffin, L., & Kolomer, S. R. (2000). Grandparent caregivers I: Characteristics of the grandparents and the children with disabilities for whom they care. *Journal of Gerontological Social Work, 33*, 35–55.

Kelley, S. J., Whitley, D. M., & Campos, P. E. (2011). Behavior problems in children raised by grandmothers: The role of caregiver distress, family resources, and the home environment. *Children and Youth Services Review, 33*, 2138–2145.

Kelley, S. J., Whitley, D. M., & Campos, P. E. (2013). Psychological distress in African American grandmothers raising grandchildren: The contribution of child behavior problems, physical health, and family resources. *Research in Nursing & Health, 36*, 373–385.

Kolomer, S. R., McCallion, P., & Janicki, M. P. (2002). African-American grandmother carers of children with disabilities: Predictors of depressive symptoms. *Journal of Gerontological Social Work, 37*, 45–63.

Kresak, K. E., Gallagher, P. A., & Kelley, S. J. (2014). Grandmothers raising grandchildren with disabilities: Sources of support and family quality of life. *Journal of Early Intervention, 36*, 3–17.

Lee, Y., & Blitz, L. V. (2014). We're GRAND: A qualitative design and development pilot project addressing the needs and strengths of grandparents raising grandchildren. *Child and Family Social Work,*. doi:10.1111/cfs.12153

Musil, C., Warner, C., Zauszniewski, J., Wykle, M., & Standing, T. (2009). Grandmother caregiving, family stress and strain, and depressive symptoms. *Western Journal of Nursing Research, 31*, 389–408.

Neely-Barnes, S. L., & Dia, D. A. (2008). Families of children with disabilities: A review of literature and recommendations for interventions. *Journal of Early and Intensive Behavior Intervention, 5*(2008), 93–107.

Rubin, M. (2013). Grandparents as caregivers: Emerging issues for the profession. *Journal of Human Behavior in the Social Environment, 23*, 330–344.

Schilmoeller, G. L., & Baranowski, M. D. (1998). Intergenerational support in families with disabilities: Grandparents' perspectives. *Families in Society, 79*, 465–476.

Shakya, H. B., Usita, P. M., Eisenberg, C., Weston, J., & Liles, S. (2012). Family well-being concerns of grandparents in skipped generation families. *Journal of Gerontological Social Work, 55*, 39–54.

Yancura, L. A. (2013). Service use and unmet service needs in grandparents raising grandchildren. *Journal of Gerontological Social Work, 56*, 473–486.

Chapter 6
A Long Way to Go—From Awareness to Practice

Professionals' Perceptions of Grandparents of Children with Disabilities

Liora Findler

Abstract Although professionals recognize the crucial contribution of grandparents to families of children with disabilities, they seldom translate this acknowledgment to practice with grandparents. This chapter presents an integrative review of studies on the perception of grandparents held by social workers, educators, pediatricians, and nurses. It relates to a variety of aspects, including the importance of the support provided to the family by the grandparents; the type of support required by the parents versus the actual support provided; the contribution of the grandparents' support to the parents' adjustment; and the costs and benefits of grandparents' involvement in the life of the nuclear family. The chapter reveals the discrepancy between professionals' acknowledgement of the importance of grandparents' contribution and their absence from programs and activities offered in practice.

Keywords Grandparenthood · Grandchildren with a disability · Professionals · Teachers · Nurses · Social workers · Physicians · Practice with grandparents of children with disabilities

Education, welfare, and healthcare professionals all recognize that the way in which a nuclear family copes with the challenges of raising a child with a disability affects the child's ability to adapt (Florian and Elad 1998; Frey et al. 1989; Quittner et al. 1992). Similarly, the way in which the extended family is involved and provides support affects the coping and adjustment of the nuclear family (Findler 2000). As a result of this understanding, professional interventions for children with disabilities have changed dramatically over the past decades, shifting from a focus exclusively on the child to a broader focus on the entire family, including the parents, siblings, and grandparents (e.g., Carroll 2013; Findler and Vardi 2009; Findler 2014). Furthermore, a new approach has become widely accepted among professionals: perception of the family of the child with a disability as a partner and ally in therapeutic and educational processes.

L. Findler and O. Taubman – Ben-Ari, *Grandparents of Children with Disabilities*, SpringerBriefs in Well-Being and Quality of Life Research,
DOI 10.1007/978-3-319-45517-4_6

This approach, dubbed Family Centered Service (FCS), a term coined by Rosenbaum et al. (1998), is based on recognition of the strengths and distinctive cultural and socio-economic identity of the family. The family is perceived as a whole, and at the same time the unique needs and qualities of each individual member is taken into consideration. Based on the premise that optimal child functioning occurs in the framework of a supportive familial and communal context, FCS regards the family as a full partner in decisions relating to the treatment and future of a child with a disability, while respecting each member of the family and his or her needs. In recent years, this model has been adopted by professionals from the realms of healthcare, education, and welfare. Studies show that parents welcome the partnership, and indeed, their contentment with professionals has found to be closely linked to the implementation of this approach. They feel they are being heard, that their input is regarded as valuable, and that their status as full partners is expressed in the receipt of information and participation in the decision-making process (King et al. 2004). These findings are not surprising, as parents often report that one of the most difficult aspects of parenting is the interaction with professionals (Hodge and Runswick-Cole 2008). Although many professionals acknowledge the merits of FCS, it will still take time for them to assimilate the approach, and it is not yet universally implemented. Furthermore, despite the fact that FCS defines the term "family" in the broad sense, the contribution of support provided by the extended family in general, and the grandparents in particular, is often overlooked.

Whether or not they adopt FCS in practice, all professionals recognize the importance of social support in reducing stress and contributing to the adjustment of the family of a child with a disability (Dunst et al. 1986; Findler 2007, 2008; Findler and Taubman – Ben-Ari 2003; Floyd and Zmich 1991). Their reports indicate that emotional support consisting of attentiveness, sympathy, understanding, and encouragement enables the parents to better express their feelings. This contributes to reducing the sense of isolation that often stems from the intensity of the child's care and the social stigma associated with disability (Dunst, Trivette, and Deal 1988). Research also points to the critical importance of instrumental support (e.g., financial support, transportation, babysitting, running errands) for parents who are coping with the challenge of raising a child with a disability (Unger and Powell 1980; Wandersman et al. 1980). Assistance may be provided both by the formal/professional system and by the informal system of family and friends. However, clinicians and decision makers tend to overlook the potential contribution of the informal support network to the physical and psychological well-being of families of children with disabilities (Dunst et al. 1988; Florian and Krulik 1991; Kazak and Wilcox 1984; Rimmerman and Stranger 1992; Seybold et al. 1991). Furthermore, studies conducted in the US (Dunst et al. 1988) and Israel (Florian and Krulik 1991; Rimmerman and Stranger 1992) show that parents of children with disabilities prefer the informal support provided by family members and friends rather than the support of professionals. This may be because informal support allows for mutuality, and thus reduces the sense of dependence and helplessness which might accompany the receipt of assistance. It is also possible that people feel more comfortable accepting help from their closest relatives, with whom they share emotional ties and a sense of solidarity.

The literature indicates that grandparents may constitute a major source of informal support in families who are coping with various kinds of stress (e.g., Baranowski and Schilmoeller 1999; Findler 2000; Seligman 1991). A number of studies have found that the contribution of grandparents in families of children with disabilities is crucial. In fact, grandparents are frequently the first to be called by the parents after they learn of their child's disability (e.g., Trute 2003; Vadasy 1987). In a study conducted among mothers of children with and without disabilities, it was found that in both groups grandparents were ranked as an important source of support (Findler 2000). Moreover, parents of children with disabilities often perceive the grandparents as a primary resource in helping to contend with the challenge of raising the child. They often report that the instrumental support provided by the grandparents (helping with the children, household chores, transportation, etc.), along with the emotional support gained by sharing the pain and exchanging information, greatly promote the family's sense of security and stability (Findler 2000).

Although their importance is recognized by professionals, grandparents are seldom included in their activities and their role is largely overlooked in the literature. This chapter reviews a series of studies, which, for the first time, examined the attitudes of professionals to the role of grandparents in families of children with disabilities. All the professionals who participated in these studies embrace the FCS model, and they include social workers, educators (school and pre-school teachers), and healthcare professionals (nurses and pediatricians). The first study examined the attitudes of 81 social workers who provided services to families of children with developmental disabilities (Findler and Taubman – Ben-Ari 2003). The second study examined 162 educators in pre-school and elementary schools, 80 of whom worked in special education (Findler 2007). The third investigation studied the perceptions of 52 pediatricians and 93 nurses in relation to the role of grandparents in families of children with an illness (Findler 2008). The chapter concludes with suggestions for a model for working with grandparents.

The three studies examined the perceptions of welfare, education, and healthcare professionals regarding various aspects of the grandparents' involvement, including: the significance of the support provided to the parents; the kind of support needed by the parents; and the kind of support which professionals deemed the grandparents actually provided. The participants were also asked to assess the contribution of the grandparents' support to the parent's adjustment, and to relate to the question of the costs and benefits of this support for the parents. Finally, the studies examined whether the professionals' attitudes are implemented in practice, their need for further information, and their willingness to learn and acquire new intervention strategies for grandparents.

6.1 Professionals' Ranking of Grandparents' Contribution

When social workers and teachers were asked to assess grandparents' contribution to families of children with disabilities, most of them described the grandparents as a stable and meaningful factor within the parents' support system. Their rankings of the grandparents' support, however, indicated significant differences in the way they perceived grandmothers versus grandfathers, and maternal versus paternal grandparents. Both social workers and teachers ranked the mother of each parent as the second source of support after the parent's spouse. The maternal grandmother was perceived as highly meaningful not only for her daughter, the mother, but also for the father. Fathers-in-law were ranked almost in the last place.

The professionals' ranking of the grandparents is in line with ranking performed by mothers, as shown in a study by Findler (2000), where mothers of children with disabilities were asked to rank the twelve people in their support network in order of importance. The mothers ranked the grandparents relatively higher than other figures, with the maternal grandmother ranked first and the maternal grandfather fifth. The paternal grandmother was ranked eighth and the paternal grandfather eleventh.

6.2 Professionals' Perceptions of Grandparents' Support

Teachers, social workers, pediatricians, and nurses all regarded the grandparents as much needed agents of emotional support, followed in descending order by instrumental and financial support, and providing information and advice. In addition, while they perceived both parents as equally in need of instrumental support, they perceived the mothers as needing more emotional support than the fathers, and the fathers as needing more financial support, information, and advice than the mothers.

Here, too, professionals and mothers' perceptions were similar in relation to the type of support required, and both ranked the grandparents' emotional support as the most significant. It is reasonable to assume that it is easier to expect emotional support from people who are closer and with whom one feels solidarity and kinship. Instrumental support, on the other hand, can also be provided by those with whom one is less intimate or by paid employees with whom the relationship is less charged. Furthermore, while grandparents' ability to provide physical and financial support might be limited by health and financial circumstances, they can still be expected to provide emotional support, encouragement, and the sense that they share in the parents' experience.

Although the three professional groups felt that the parents needed more emotional support than instrumental, they indicated that more instrumental support was actually being provided. All professionals perceived the support offered by grandparents to be high, and all of them believed it was essentially instrumental, followed in descending order by emotional support, financial support, and information and advice. In regard to this issue, the professionals' views are not consistent with the findings of most studies on parents, who report receiving more emotional than instrumental support from the grandparents (Findler 2000; Hornby and Ashworth 1994; Trute 2003; Trute et al. 2008). Two earlier studies, however, yielded contrasting results that are more in line with the perceptions of the professionals. Seybold et al. (1991) found that parents of children with disabilities received more instrumental than emotional support from the grandparents. Heller et al. (2000), who asked mothers about grandparents' support at three phases in the child's life cycle (childhood, adolescence, and adulthood) found that grandparents provided their children with more instrumental support in the first phase than in the later ones.

When ranking the grandparents' contribution to the adjustment of each parent, all three groups of professionals deemed that they generally contributed more to the mother's adjustment than to the father's on all dimensions. In addition, they believed that grandparents' involvement contributed primarily to emotional and parental adaptation, and to a lesser extent to marital, social, and occupational adaptation. Only the teachers indicated no differences between mothers and fathers in relation to marital life, which they ranked last after the contribution to emotional and parental adaptation.

6.3 Costs and Benefits of Grandparents' Involvement as Perceived by Professionals

Professionals' views regarding the costs and benefits to the parents of grandparents' support were expressed in answers to open questions. On the whole, they referred to their instrumental and emotional support as beneficial. More specifically, they referred to the value of the grandparents' participation in activities such as trips, meals, and family celebrations, and described the emotional support provided by the grandparents in terms such as attentiveness, care, and encouragement. The teachers thought that the grandparents were more sensitive and attentive to the parents' feelings and needs than any other member of their support network. Nevertheless, conflicts and difficulties were also mentioned, although less frequently. A few teachers felt that grandparents themselves could become a source of stress when they blamed their children for the grandchild's disability and criticized their parenting. They also expressed their belief that some grandparents fail to understand the child's special needs or to empathize with the challenges of raising a child with a disability.

The themes emerging from the answers of pediatricians and nurses referred both to the instrumental and the emotional support provided during treatment of a sick child. Similar to the teachers, they considered the grandparents to be more sensitive and attentive to the parents' feelings and needs than any other member of their social network. They spoke of intergenerational solidarity and a sense of commitment, as well as grandparents' participation in the decision making process and the gathering of information with regard to treatment, rights, and available services. Although the health professionals referred less to the costs of grandparents' involvement than the teachers, their reports covered a wider range of topics. The cost most often mentioned was the strain and stress on parents due to grandparents' over-involvement, anxieties, and lack of faith in the parents' capabilities. They also referred to intergenerational gaps, archaic or irrelevant ideas on the part of the grandparents, excessive involvement and interference throughout the course of treatment, inappropriate emotional reactions, and the parents' reluctance to share medical information with the grandparents.

By virtue of their work, social workers are more used to engaging in conversations with family members on disturbing issues, such as the costs and benefits of the grandparents' support, than other professionals. Overall, the social workers depicted grandparents as a stable and significant component of the social support network of parents of children with disabilities. However, they elaborated more on the costs of the grandparents' involvement than the other professional groups. Five categories of costs were listed: disappointment with the minimal instrumental support offered by the grandparents; disappointment with the grandparents' emotional support (indifference, inattentiveness, lack of knowledge or caring); over-involvement in the life of the nuclear family (criticizing the couple's relationship, blaming the parents for the child's condition, establishing a coalition with one parent against the other); negative attitudes toward the child with the disability (shame, disappointment, rejection, avoidance, favoring one grandchild over others); lack of knowledge and skills in coping with the special needs of the child (over-protectiveness).

Despite the commonalities among the professionals, their responses varied as a result of their different professional perceptions and the nature of their relationship with the family. While education and health care professionals focused on the child, social workers focused mainly on the family; whereas teachers, pediatricians, and nurses reported their impressions of the families from random encounters, social workers dedicated a part of their sessions with the parents to family issues in general, and the grandparents' role in particular. Consequently, different issues came to the fore in each group of professionals in respect to the difficulties in the relationship with the grandparents.

Negative aspects of grandparents' involvement also appear in the literature from the perspective of the parents. Thus, for example, the gap between the parents' perceptions and that of the grandparents regarding the child's condition and future prognosis may be a source of tension and anger for the parents. These reactions are aggravated when the parents sense denial of the child's disability on the part of the grandparents. This implies lack of acceptance of the child as he or she is on the one hand, and lack of acknowledgment of the special needs of both the child and the parents on the other (Seligman 1991; Seligman et al. 1997). According to Seligman (1991) and George (1988), parents might get caught up in stressful situations when grandparents' failure to understand the nature of the child's disability leads to doubt as to the need for special treatment programs. This sort of overly optimistic approach, which assumes that "things will work themselves out", is occasionally accompanied by attitudes of hostility, confusion, avoidance, fear, or shame toward the child, increasing the tension with the parents. Moreover, parents often report more tension and conflicts with the paternal grandparents than with the maternal grandparents (Hornby and Ashworth 1994).

6.4 Professionals' Interactions with the Grandparents

The teachers' replies showed that they were fully aware of the importance of the grandparents' role. This understanding, however, was not always implemented in practice. Most teachers reported that they seldom met with any of the grandparents and that they saw paternal grandparents less than maternal grandparents. When meetings did take place, they were initiated mostly by the parents, grandparents, or other professionals, and not by the teachers themselves. Importantly, most teachers stated that they had no interest in special training to improve their skills and knowledge with regard to grandparents.

Similarly, the majority of social workers believed that involving the grandparents in interventions for families of children with disabilities was only rarely appropriate, and noted that by law, approaching other family members is subject to the parents' consent. Grandparents are not normally included in such interventions for a variety of reasons, such as a strained relationship between the generations, the wish to protect the grandparents due to their poor health or advanced age, and, on occasion, parents' desire to be exclusively responsible for the care of the child. When grandparents are included, the parents are also present. Most social workers reported having seldom met with grandparents, and then it was more likely to be with the maternal grandparents than with the paternal grandparents. Furthermore, only a quarter of these meetings were initiated by the social workers themselves, and the rest by either the parents or the grandparents. Approximately half of the social workers stated that they were not interested in any special training or courses aimed at improving their skills and knowledge in respect to grandparents.

In contrast, most of the pediatricians, and even a greater number of the nurses, had often met the grandparents, but only when they escorted the grandchild to treatment. Again, in most cases these meetings were initiated by the parents, grandparents, or other professionals, and not by the healthcare professionals themselves. Like the other groups, most nurses, and even more pediatricians, indicated that they were not interested in any special training or courses to improve their skills and knowledge in relation to grandparents.

To conclude, although professionals in the fields of education, welfare, and healthcare recognize the importance of grandparents' involvement and their contribution to various domains, they rarely initiate meetings or interact with them. Most notably, they have little interest in expanding their skills and knowledge in the matter. Moreover, Professionals' reports raise many issues regarding the role of grandparents in the family, their contribution to the parents' well-being, the nature of their contribution and the costs and benefits of their support. Nonetheless, they rarely mention grandparents' emotional experience with respect to the grandchild's disability and its impact on their lives.

Despite the growth in individual and group activities for grandparents of children with disabilities, they remain sporadic and exist only as part of the services for the children and their parents. In other words, there is a discrepancy between professionals' acknowledgement of the importance of grandparents' contribution and the programs offered for or about them in practice.

Grandparents display a variety of distinctive and diverse responses, come to terms with the situation at different paces, and employ disparate coping methods, making it incumbent on professionals to choose the most suitable approach for each of them, be it individual, family, or group therapy. Moreover, even professionals who do not interact with the grandparents directly can discuss with the parents the relationship with the grandparents and ways to benefit from their potential contribution.

There is no doubt that grandparents can be an important source of support for families of children with disabilities, as they not only have life experience, but are also likely to have the time, motivation, and commitment to provide emotional and instrumental support (Gardner et al. 1994; Seligman 1991; Seligman et al. 1997). Nonetheless, little has been done to make the most of this potential. By creating a partnership between professionals and the parents, FCS has dramatically changed the approach of professionals, including those who participated in these studies. However, their focus remains on the nuclear, rather than the extended, family.

Another approach, called the Family Systems Illness model (FSI) (Rolland 1994), seeks to broaden the focus to include the extended family in general, and the intergenerational relationship in particular. According to the FSI, which deals, *inter alia*, with multigenerational patterns of coping with illness and loss, the fact that the child's disability will forever be part of the family's life heightens the necessity to relate to the needs of each of the family members, and not only to those of the child. As a result of imbalance or total disregard for these needs, the members of the extended family may not only fail to serve as a source of support for the child and the nuclear family, but may even become a source of further distress. Rolland (1994) contends that professionals should initiate a professional dialogue with all members of the extended family at a very early stage to avoid the conflicts, tension, disparities in expectations, and communication problems that may emerge later, when they will require elaborate interventions.

Various intervention strategies may be effective for grandparents of children with disabilities, including individual therapy, family therapy, or e-therapy. The experience gained thus far indicates that group counselling may provide a good response to the needs of many grandparents. The presence of other people who have had or are now having similar experiences offers them the opportunity to express their feelings, gives these feelings legitimacy, and creates an affiliation group, which affords reliable and sensitive support.

Existing programs for these grandparents generally set the following goals (e.g., Pacer n.d.; Beit issie Shapiro):

- To enable grandparents of children with disabilities to meet other grandparents in a similar situation and share common feelings and interests;
- To provide grandparents with emotional support and legitimacy for the disturbing feelings they might experience, such as disappointment, anxiety, anger, ambivalence, frustration, etc.;
- To provide grandparents with an understanding of the nature, etiology, and prognosis of the disability, as well as with details of the sources of information, services, and organizations available to them;
- To help to improve the relationship with the nuclear family, set realistic expectations, establish a division of roles, and open channels of communication between the generations;
- To provide an opportunity for the grandparents to practice skills relating specifically to the child's development and unique needs.

It is important to remember that interventions for grandparents will be of little value if they exist in a vacuum. Professionals must work simultaneously with the parents in order to create a productive give-and-take in respect to expectations, division of roles, and communication.

Currently, there is no coherent policy regarding the grandparents of children with disabilities, and in most countries, the package of services for these children makes no mention of grandparents. Given these circumstances, intervention programs for grandparents are subject to the discretion and initiative of professionals or organizations, and as such they are sporadic and unsystematic.

It is imperative that the growing acknowledgement of the importance of grandparents' support in families of children with disabilities be given practical form. This requires the formulation of policy guidelines and the allocation of resources to the development of training programs for working with the extended family, and grandparents in particular. Once such programs are integrated into the curricula of Schools of Education, Social Work, Public Health, and Medicine, professionals' awareness of the significance of intergenerational relationships in families of children with disabilities will be greatly enhanced, undoubtedly giving rise to interventions aimed at realizing the full potential of the grandparents for the benefit of all family members.

References

Baranowski, M., & Schilmoeller, G. L. (1999). Grandparents in the lives of grandchildren with disabilities: Mothers' perceptions. *Education and Treatment of Children, 22*, 427–446.

Beit Issie Shapiro, Early Intervention Center. Retreived from http://en.beitissie.org.il/about/early-intervention

Carroll, D. W. (2013). Initial experience and reactions. In D. W. Carroll (Ed.), *Families of children with developmental disabilities: Understanding stress and opportunities for growth* (pp. 17–30). Washington, DC: American Psychological Association.

Dunst, C. J., Trivette, C. M., & Cross, A. H. (1986). Mediating influences of social support: Personal, family, and child outcomes. *American Journal of Mental Deficiency, 90*, 403–417.
Dunst, C. J., Trivette, C. M., & Deal, A. G. (1988). *Enabling and empowering families: Principles and guidelines for practice*. Cambridge, MA: Brookline Books.
Findler, L. (2007). Grandparents—The overlooked potential partners: Perceptions and practice of teachers in special and regular education. *European Journal of Special Needs Education, 22*, 199–216.
Findler, L. (2008). Support behind the scenes: Attitudes and practice of pediatricians and nurses with grandparents of sick children. *Family, Community and Health: The Journal of Health Promotion & Maintenance, 31*, 317–325.
Findler, L. (2014). The experience of stress and personal growth among grandparents of children with and without intellectual disability. *Intellectual and Developmental Disabilities, 52*, 32–48.
Findler, L. S. (2000). The role of grandparents in the social support system of mothers of children with a physical disability. *Families in Society, 81*, 370–381.
Findler, L., & Taubman – Ben-Ari, O. (2003). Social workers' perceptions and practice regarding grandparents in families of children with a developmental disability. *Families in Society, 84*, 86–94.
Findler, L., & Vardi, A. (2009). Psychological growth among siblings of children with and without intellectual disabilities. *Intellectual and Developmental Disabilities, 47*, 1–12.
Florian, V., & Elad, D. (1998). The impact of mothers' sense of empowerment on the metabolic control of their children with juvenile diabetes. *Journal of Pediatric Psychology, 23*, 239–247.
Florian, V., & Krulik, T. (1991). Loneliness and social support of mothers of chronically ill children. *Social Science and Medicine, 32*, 1291–1296.
Floyd, F. J., & Zmich, D. E. (1991). Marriage and the parenting partnership: Perceptions and interactions of parents with mentally retarded and typically developing children. *Child Development, 62*, 1434–1448.
Frey, K. S., Fewell, R. R., & Vadasy, P. F. (1989). Parental adjustment and changes in child outcome among families of young handicapped children. *Topics in Early Childhood Special Education, 8*, 38–57.
Gardner, J. E., Scherman, A., Mobley, D., Brown, P., & Schutter, M. (1994). Grandparents' beliefs regarding their role and relationship with special needs grandchildren. *Education and Treatment of Children, 17*, 185–196.
George, J. D. (1988). Therapeutic intervention for grandparents and extended family of children with developmental delays. *Mental Retardation, 26*, 369–375.
Heller, T., Heish, K., & Rowitz, L. (2000). Grandparents as supports to mothers of persons with intellectual disability. *Journal of Gerontological Social Work, 33*, 23–34.
Hodge, N., & Runswick-Cole, K. (2008). Problematising parent-professional partnerships in education. *Disability & Society, 23*, 637–647.
Hornby, G., & Ashworth, T. (1994). Grandparents' support for families who have children with disabilities. *Journal of Child and Family Studies, 3*, 403–412.
Kazak, A. E., & Wilcox, B. L. (1984). The structure and function of social support networks in families with handicapped children. *American Journal of Community Psychology, 12*, 645–661.
King, S., Teplicky, R., King, G., & Rosenbaum, P. (2004). Family centered service for children with cerebral palsy and their families: A review of the literature. *Seminars in Pediatric Neurology, 11*, 78–86.
Pacer. (n.d). Grandparent to grandparent program overview. Retrieved from http://www.pacer.org/grandparent/
Quittner, A. L., DiGirolamo, A. M., Michel, M., & Eigen, H. (1992). Parental response to cystic fibrosis: A contextual analysis of the diagnosis phase. *Journal of Pediatric Psychology, 17*, 683–704.
Rimmerman, A., & Stranger, V. (1992). Locus of control and utilization of social support among mothers of young children with physical disabilities. *International Journal of Rehabilitation Research, 15*, 39–48.

Rolland, J. S. (1994). *Families, illness and disability; An integrative treatment model*. New York, NY: Basic Books.

Rosenbaum, P., King, S., Law, M., King, G., & Evans, J. (1998). Family-centred service: A conceptual framework and research review. *Physical & Occupational Therapy in Pediatrics, 18*, 1–20.

Seligman, M. (1991). Grandparents of disabled grandchildren: Hopes, fears, and adaptation. *Families in Society, 72*, 147–152.

Seligman, M., Goodwin, G., Paschal, K., Applegate, A., & Lehman, L. (1997). Grandparents of children with disabilities: Perceived levels of support. *Education and Training in Mental Retardation and Developmental Disabilities, 32*, 293–303.

Seybold, J., Fritz, J., & MacPhee, D. (1991). Relation of social support to the self-perceptions of mothers with delayed children. *Journal of Community Psychology, 19*, 29–36.

Trute, B. (2003). Grandparents of children with developmental disabilities: Intergenerational support and family well-being. *Families in Society, 84*, 119–126.

Trute, B., Worthington, C., & Hiebert-Murphy, D. (2008). Grandmother support for parents of children with disabilities: Gender differences in parenting stress. *Families, Systems, & Health, 26*, 135–146.

Unger, D. G., & Powell, D. R. (1980). Supporting families under stress: The role of social networks. *Family Relations, 29*, 566–574.

Vadasy, P. F. (1987). Grandparents of children with special needs: Supports especially for grandparents. *Children's Health Care, 16*, 21–23.

Wandersman, L. P., Wandersman, A., & Kahn, S. (1980). Social support in the transition to parenthood. *Journal of Community Psychology, 8*, 332–342.

Final Words: From Behind the Scene to Front Stage—Learning from the Past and Looking to the Future

Orit Taubman - Ben-Ari and Liora Findler

Grandparenthood is one of the most significant roles in adult life, second only to the role of parent. Nevertheless, over the years it has received only marginal research attention. This book is part of the effort to alter that reality and encourage discussion, investigation, and clinical intervention initiatives devoted to grandparents.

A survey of the historical development of the grandparent role reveals how external changes, including increased longevity and modifications in the structure of the traditional family, have given it new meaning. Moreover, the transition to grandparenthood inevitably triggers internal changes, adding a new element to the factors that define the individual's personal and family identity. In both the internal and external contexts, the role involves a diversity of facets on a variety of levels, and as such, may arouse not only positive emotions, but also stress and distress that may come into play in the wake of certain events or circumstances.

Creating a new family requires melding together the disparate worlds of norms, behaviors, and values of the two families of origin and of different generations. While the process may afford a sense of unity and solidarity, it is also fraught with sensitivities, incompatible attitudes, unresolved issues from the past, and breakdowns in communication, all of which may lead to conflict, anger, and frustration. In particularly unique circumstances, such as the birth of a child with a disability, the vulnerability of the family system is even greater, and may also be reflected in intergenerational relationships. The question of support from the extended family in general, and the grandparents in particular, is liable to become a central and ongoing issue in relations between the middle generation, that is, the child's parents, and the grandparents.

With people now living longer, it is not unusual for a child to have three or four living grandparents. Thus grandparents may represent a large proportion of the family and may have a critical impact on it. Their presence in the fabric of the nuclear family may fall anywhere along the spectrum from supportive and benevolent to stressful and frustrating. Yet grandparents' potential to be a major factor in the family's informal support system, particularly in the case of the family of a child with disabilities, has not received the attention it deserves, either in the research literature or in clinical practice. This may be a reflection of the attitude of parents and professionals, and perhaps of grandparents themselves. Grandparents are typically

L. Findler and O. Taubman - Ben-Ari, *Grandparents of Children with Disabilities*,
SpringerBriefs in Well-Being and Quality of Life Research,
DOI 10.1007/978-3-319-45517-4

assessed solely on the functional level, that is, by the degree of instrumental support they provide for their children and grandchildren, with no regard for other aspects of the role, including their own experience of grandparenthood and the implications of being the grandparent of a child with a disability.

This book looks at grandparents from a wide range of angles, shedding light on the processes, experiences, and responses of grandparents themselves, while also exposing the scarcity of research and clinical knowledge of this population. The studies presented here, along with the remarks drawn from interviews with grandparents, make it clear that grandparents want their voice to be heard and wish to share their experiences and feelings. They repeatedly expressed gratitude to the researchers for taking an interest in them and for the importance they attributed to their role. Interviews with grandparents of children with disabilities, in particular, elicited several themes of distinct significance to them, including: the shock of learning about the child's disability; the process of coming to terms with the disability; their relations with their children in light of the expectation, or demand, for their support; the delicate balance between involvement and interference in the life of the nuclear family; the costs and benefits associated with providing, or not providing, support; and the lack of response to their own needs from formal frameworks or professionals, along with the absence a clinical programs or guidance designed for grandparents.

Another issue addressed in this book is the growing phenomenon of grandparents as primary caregivers of a child with a disability, and the heavy toll it takes in terms of physical health, psychological well-being, the couple relationship, and financial resources. Such grandparents face a much greater challenge than most, as they must contend not only with the implications of the life transition, but also with the absence of their own children (whether due to addiction, disease, or death), the disability of the grandchild, and the loss of their personal freedom. Even those who devote themselves and their resources unstintingly to this task and fulfill it to the very best of their ability report difficulties deriving from the lack of a formal support system designed specifically for people in their situation. In addition, they also express fear of applying for formal assistance and thereby running the risk that their competence to function as primary caretakers will be called into question and the child will be taken from them.

The book also examines the attitude of parents of children with a disability to the grandparents' support and its value for their emotional and familial well-being. It would appear that most parents consider the contribution of the grandparents' emotional support to be greater than that of their instrumental support. On the other hand, disparities between the parents and grandparents in regard to assessment of the child's condition, expectations pertaining to help and support, or the desirable degree of involvement in the life of the nuclear family are often the source of tension and conflict between the two generations. In addition, the book presents the attitudes of another group of major relevance that is almost totally ignored in the literature: professionals in the fields of medicine, social work, and education. The series of studies examining professionals' perceptions of grandparents' potential to constitute a major resource for the family of a child with a disability reveals the gap between existing knowledge and its translation into actual practice, between acknowledgement of the importance of grandparents' support and their absence from clinical and guidance programs for such families.

While the book paints a broad picture of intergenerational relationships in families of children with a disability, it also raises issues that demand further and more comprehensive investigation. These include, for example: the grandchild's attitude toward the grandparents; changes over time in intergenerational relationships as the various family members grow older and the balance of power between them is altered; differences in the attitudes and perceptions of mothers and fathers, grandmothers and grandfathers, and maternal and paternal grandparents in view of the child's disability; the role of grandparents in single-parent and single-sex families of a child with a disability; the place of great-grandparents in the family; and the grandparent role in families of children with a disability in different cultures.

It is our hope that this book will encourage policy-makers to institute clear and standardized procedures for the allocation of resources to enhancing intergenerational relations, and that professionals will develop dedicated intervention methods for parents and grandparents aimed at realizing the huge potential of this natural resource. With such efforts in place, the crucial role of grandparents in the family is likely to become part of the social consciousness, paving the way for recognition of the total experience of grandparenthood and the emotional and psychological processes the individual undergoes with the birth of a grandchild in general, and a grandchild with a disability in particular. Our ultimate vision is that from the start of socialization and in each and every training program for the pertinent professionals, intergenerational relationships in the family and the unique role of the grandparents will receive the attention they warrant. Professionals who understand the importance of this issue will be able to use the knowledge they have gained to develop dedicated programs and courses for grandparents, helping all generations to benefit from this exceptional family resource.